MAX FRENCH
HANNAH HESSELGREAV
ROB WILSON
MELISSA HAWKINS
TOBY LOWE

HARNESSING COMPLEXITY FOR BETTER OUTCOMES IN PUBLIC AND NON-PROFIT SERVICES

POLICY PRESS SHORTS POLICY & PRACTICE

First published in Great Britain in 2023 by

Policy Press, an imprint of
Bristol University Press
University of Bristol
1-9 Old Park Hill
Bristol
BS2 8BB
UK
t: +44 (0)117 374 6645
e: bup-info@bristol.ac.uk

Details of international sales and distribution partners are available at
policy.bristoluniversitypress.co.uk

British Library Cataloguing in Publication Data
A catalogue record for this book is available from the British Library

ISBN 978-1-4473-6411-5 paperback
ISBN 978-1-4473-6412-2 ePub
ISBN 978-1-4473-6413-9 OA PDF

To Beatrice, James H, James W, Marin, Alistair,
Noah, Grace, and Fleur

Contents

List of figures and tables

Figures

Tables

About the authors

Max French is Lecturer in Systems Leadership at Northumbria University. Max's academic background is grounded in research partnerships with charitable foundations, governments, and civil society organisations. His research focus and recent outputs are centred on four overlapping areas: the governance of complexity in public services, the role of outcomes in policymaking and public administration, action-oriented research approaches, and transitions toward sustainable development and collective wellbeing.

Hannah Hesselgreaves is Professor of Organisational Learning at Northumbria University. With a background in organisational psychology, she has developed a portfolio of work in the areas of learning transfer (and the evaluation of outcomes), job quality, and employee wellbeing. Her research is aimed at informing policy and practice in the workplace, including interprofessional education, collaborative learning, and learning partnering in public service contexts. Hannah also founded her own research company and has driven many research and consultancy projects commissioned across the public and voluntary and community sector (VCS), including work with Joseph Rowntree Trust.

Rob Wilson is Professor of Digital Economy at Northumbria University has over two decades of experience working on and leading public service information systems/digital government research and development projects. His work is based in three overlapping contexts – the integration and information aspects of public services (in particular contexts of health and social care – including children, older people and families); the challenges of technology adoption, data, information, and measurement in local governance and the role of information and information systems. His research is covered in two recent books, *Digital Government @ Work* (Oxford University Press, 2013) and *Digital Disruption and the Digitalisation of Healthcare* (Oxford University Press, 2017).

Melissa Hawkins is Lecturer at Northumbria University and started her career in education, working as a classroom teacher in schools for nine years. She then moved to higher education where she acted as a teaching fellow in academic skills and learning development at two universities in the South West of England. Her PhD research applies complexity theory as a theoretical framework to problematise performance management in schools. Until recently she has been working on action-oriented research projects, focused on the development of complexity-informed public management practice, including the role of engaged scholarship in learning partnerships.

Toby Lowe is Assistant Professor in Public Management at Northumbria University and currently on Secondment as Visiting Professor to the Centre for Public Impact (CPI) an international Social Enterprise whose aim is to transform government. Before rejoining academia he had a number of roles including working as a Civil Servant on place-based regeneration projects and as Chief Executive of an Arts-based charity working with people with complex needs. His main focus is the development of theory and practice of Human Learning Systems (HLS), an alternative approach to orthodox approaches to public management. He has produced a number of publications on HLS, including most recently the Practical User guide for the Curious.

Acknowledgements

We would like to express our gratitude for the support, guidance, and patience of the team at Policy Press and our reviewers.

It has been an enduring privilege to work with our friends and collaborators in a wide range of shared adventures related to this book's topic. These have been foundational to the insights presented in this text. This book is also a product of its five authors' different perspectives. We take responsibility for any inconsistencies which may have arisen, but consider these a worthwhile sacrifice for a book which is more than the sum of its parts. This is the end of the beginning of a journey, and there is still much more to do.

Preface

Who can remember a more challenging time to be a public servant?

From global heating to demographic change to entrenching social inequalities, a growing cast of wicked issues demand bold new policy agendas stretching years, if not decades, into the future. Sudden 'black swan' shocks from climate emergencies to global pandemics demand the opposite: immediate, game-changing adaptation. Fiscal retrenchment in recent years has reduced the capacity of many nation states to respond to either challenge, while declining trust in governments and public organisations now sets citizens at odds with the institutions designed to serve them. Looking forward, the only thing we might accurately predict is yet more uncertainty.

This book tackles a problem animating policymakers, service professionals, and academics alike: in an increasingly complex world, how can public services and social interventions create and sustain positive outcomes for the people and populations they serve?

We argue for a radical change in the form and function of public administration and governance. Genuine social outcomes – those high-level conditions of societal wellbeing like quality-of-life, health, criminal behaviour, or educational attainment – are simply too complex to be delivered by top-down policymaking, target-driven management, contractualism, or more rigorously-evidenced social interventions. Outcomes across the human and relational services are better achieved and value better created by investing in the capability of public service systems to engage meaningfully with the complexity of people's lives.

Building from foundational scholarship in public health, we develop an alternative theoretical perspective on value creation in the public sector. Our Complexity Theory of Outcome Creation (CTOC) explains how complex dynamics shape how outcomes emerge within individuals and embed across populations. We use this as a design guide to set out an alternative agenda for public service reform across the human and relational services.

We present a critical analysis of two pragmatic and accessible practices currently engaging academics and researchers in this agenda: Human Learning Systems, a leading collaborative endeavour into complexity-informed public service reform, and learning partnerships, an action-oriented model for research and academic engagement in complex settings.

This book draws together insight won from a decade of engaged scholarship with policymakers and practitioners (Lowe 2013; French 2014; 2017; Lowe et al 2016; Lowe and Wilson 2017; French and Lowe 2018; Lowe et al 2020a; 2020b; French et al 2021a; French and Mollinger-Sahba 2021; Lowe et al 2021b; Hesselgreaves et al 2021; French et al 2022; Wilson et al in press), policy-oriented research (Pell et al 2016; Davidson-Knight et al 2017; Lowe and French 2018; Lowe and Plimmer 2019, Pell et al 2020; Lowe et al 2021b; French et al in press; Lowe et al 2022), alongside new empirical material, into a cohesive and authoritative contribution.

While this is an academic book, we hope it remains accessible for interested practitioners, changemakers, students, and observers. We provide a focussed and accessible examination of complexity theory in the policy and management arena but refrain from broader academic discussion. Those interested in further reading can find excellent contributions from Gerrits (2012), Byrne and Callaghan (2014), Haynes (2015), Boulton et al (2015), Jackson (2019), Harrison and Geyer (2022), and

Mowles and Norman (2022). This book is not a 'how to' guide – interested practitioners might consult Hobbs (2019) or the HLS practical guide (Lowe et al 2022) for detail on relevant applied methods. Our hope instead is to provide *terra firma* for change-oriented service professionals, policymakers, and researchers to collaborate productively, proactively, and critically with an important public service reform trajectory.

Our broad conclusions – that public service should be more relational, more responsive, better integrated, and better resourced – echo, and we hope support, various parallel streams in progressive service reform thinking (for example Elvidge 2013; Muir 2014; Needham and Mangan 2016; Cottam 2018; Lent and Studdert 2019; New Systems Alliance 2020). We end the book not with a new model or list of recommendations to adopt, but with a broad and inclusive research agenda which we hope connects together those working in research and practice in a shared learning endeavour in years to come.

This book should hold value for policymakers, practitioners, academics, and observers interested in the future of public service. Readers seeking to understand how complexity challenges the prevailing orthodoxy of public management and offers a distinctive public service reform trajectory can find our core theoretical contributions in Chapters 2, 3, and 4. Readers seeking practical insights for public service reform can consult Chapter 5 on Human Learning Systems, while those seeking to connect the worlds of research, consultancy, and practice may find Chapter 6 on learning partnerships of most interest. For readers interested in advancing knowledge, or in taking a necessary critical voice to keep this movement humble, informed, and honest, Chapter 7 sets out what we believe are the key questions which require further thought.

ONE

Introduction

In an increasingly complex world, how can public services and social interventions create value and sustain positive social outcomes for the people and populations they serve?

The orthodox response has been to optimise efficiency by sweating assets, tightening performance management structures, increasing competition, and reorienting resources from less to more productive policy interventions through identifying and scaling 'what works'. Confounding this logic is an additional threat to public service sustainability: the failure of a generation of reforms focussed on markets and competition (Le Grand 2009), targets and terror (Coulson 2009), or naming and shaming (Bevan and Wilson 2013) to improve outcomes on anything approaching a consistent basis, while often achieving something resembling the very opposite (van Thiel and Leeuw 2002; Pollitt 2013; Hood and Dixon 2016).

The reason for this failure, we argue, is that genuine social outcomes are complex phenomena which are lived by people, not delivered by public services. We devote a large section of this book to justifying this statement and considering its implications. In so doing we take in a wide-ranging exploration of academic literature spanning several disciplines over a number of decades, and survey a broad range of leading service reform practices. All that is to come — perhaps though our point can be better understood by opening a window into the world of public service. The following is a story of one public service interaction in a UK local authority.

Amy (name changed), a single parent living with her two children in social housing within a UK city, has not paid her council tax (a local services tax administered by the local authority) for two months. A notification is triggered on the computer screen of Alex, the dedicated local manager of the council's tax recovery team. In years previous, this used to trigger an escalating process of threats and sanctions to coerce payment, involving council officers, bailiffs, and eventually the criminal justice system, all at increasing expense to the taxpayer. Alex instead calls to find out why Amy hasn't paid.

Amy works part-time on a low income, and while entitled to Housing Benefit (a UK means-tested subsidy for housing costs) is above the threshold to claim council tax support. She tells Alex her payment problems began a year earlier when she split up with her partner, and found herself struggling to afford living costs by herself. Amy's grandmother, who had raised her after her mother died when she was young, had taken ill and died around the same time. She had received medical intervention and struggled to prioritise the payment of her bills.

Amy tells Alex she approached the council for help during this period, however her interactions left her with the impression: "you got into this mess, now get yourself out of it". Alex asks Amy what she thought when he requested a phonecall. She thought it was "dodgy", she said, "the council never want to help people, they just want to get their money any way they can."

Alex conducted over 30 of these conversations, carefully documenting each individual story. He found a consistent narrative. People would be passed around between specialised agencies, failing at each stage to be listened to, then eventually withdraw from service engagement. The interaction between individuals and services would often make things worse rather than better. But what would a good service interaction have looked like? This was more difficult to assess. Amy's case was influenced by a range of factors – family circumstances, mental health, relationship breakdowns, council tax policies, service access criteria. In the other cases Alex documented a huge range of disparate issues and particular factors were significant in determining non-payment: broken washing machines, anti-social behaviour from neighbours, caring duties for children, or even, in one case, pets.

Pandemics, macroeconomics, and climate catastrophe might animate contemporary policymaking, but in Alex's experience it was a multitude of particular individual factors – lived and felt most immediately – which were driving negative outcomes. What was called for was not revolutionary thinking or high-level policy change – merely empathic, flexible, holistic support – and someone to listen.

Our starting point in this book is to ask, how can we use our understanding of how outcomes emerge and embed to redesign how services operate and social interventions are managed? We will build on foundational research in public health, social epidemiology, and social determinants of health theory (Gatrell 2005; Pearce and Merletti 2006; Curtis and Riva 2010; Diez Roux 2011; Finegood 2011; Jayasinghe 2011, 2015; Rutter et al 2017), up until now neglected in public policy and public administration scholarship, to develop an alternative theoretical perspective which we call the Complexity Theory of Outcome Creation (CTOC). While this model is intuitive, we argue it directs towards a radical change of course in practice.

At the core of this is a particular theoretical understanding of how outcomes emerge at the intersection of complex lives and complex public service systems. We consider that root causes of social outcomes are multifarious and interconnected (compositional complexity), that the contributing factors, valuation, and meaning of outcomes is experienced differently from individual to individual (experiential complexity), that all these factors vary over time (dynamic complexity), and that to tackle meaningfully at scale, the multiple resources and knowledge of many different actors must be integrated into sustainable, flexible, and tailored solutions (governance complexity). Perhaps the closest visual representation might be the Penrose tile pattern, illustrated on the cover of this book. Take a minute to look at this again and try to make sense of it. The structure of the pattern collapses on closer inspection into disorder. Developed by mathematician Roger Penrose, the Penrose pattern depicts a beautiful, non-repeating structure of infinite variation – a poetic analogy for much public service work.

We show how this theoretical understanding confounds public management orthodoxy and the dominant Rationalist Theory of Outcome Creation (RTOC), which has entrenched through the new public management (NPM) reforms of the 1980s to 2000s and persisted into the current fragmented landscape of 'governance' through innovations like outcome-based contracting, social impact bonds, and other outcome-based social investment vehicles. We then transpose our CTOC into a constructive basis for public service reform and, drawing from Teece et al's (1997) theory of dynamic capabilities, set out a new research agenda in the policy and administrative sciences: building complexity-capable public services.

The book is structured as follows.

In Chapter 2, we describe how the RTOC became public management orthodoxy through the NPM reforms of the 1980s and 1990s and has persisted into the current fragmented 'governance' (Rhodes 1997) landscape through innovations like social investment vehicles, social impact bonds, outcome funds, and outcomes marketplaces. We show how, despite promising greater accountability, incentive systems, and better evidence for managerial decision making, this approach has delivered the opposite: gaming, tunnel-vision, and the destruction of morale and adaptability in public institutions.

Chapter 3 develops our alternative CTOC which builds on foundational research in public health scholarship into the emergence of population-level outcomes. We extend this model from a perspective of general complexity (Morin 2006; Byrne and Callaghan 2014) to argue that outcome complexity is foremost an issue for public administration (the financing, governance, and management of public service), not public policy.

In Chapter 4, we transpose the CTOC into pragmatic design parameters for public service reform. We draw from Teece et al's (1997) theory of dynamic capabilities to distil three core capabilities necessary in tackling this new conceptualisation of outcomes: stewardship capability, coordination capability, and adaptive capability. We argue that investment in these capabilities in consort could inform an alternative logic of outcome-focussed service reform.

In Chapter 5, we show how one avenue to operationalising a complexity-informed approach to public service reform, Human Learning Systems (HLS) (Lowe and Plimmer 2019; Hesselgreaves et al 2021; Lowe et al 2021a), has gained particular traction in policy and practitioner communities. HLS carries forward a consistent response to our CTOC, and offers an accessible design language to socialise practitioners in this logic. This critical analysis also illustrates how building complexity-capable public service institutions is difficult, long-term, and uncertain work.

Chapter 6 considers how research might support the construction of complexity-capable public services, and critically examines a 'learning partnership' approach to collaboration between academics and practitioners. We draw from two substantive learning partnerships with UK charitable foundations, Lankelly Chase Foundation and The Tudor Trust, to elaborate on how this modality of research approach can help organisations to build the necessary dynamic capabilities to cope with complexity.

In Chapter 7 we set out five organising questions which might motivate a deeper critical engagement among researchers and practitioners with building complexity-capable public services. This provides substantive material for practitioners, policymakers, and policy advocacy groups, to engage productively and critically with a new service reform trajectory.

TWO

Rationalism: a failed logic for public service reform?

The number and complexity of the problems require that we possess technical instruments of verification. But this involves two risks. We can rest content with the bureaucratic exercise of drawing up long lists of good proposals – goals, objectives and statistics – or we can think that a single theoretical and aprioristic solution will provide an answer to all the challenges.

Pope Francis' speech to the United Nations
25 September 2015 (Benedict XVI 2015)

It is now taken for granted that public services and social interventions should be financed, managed, and evaluated based on their contribution to target outcomes. In this chapter we chart the evolution of the 'outcomes imperative' in public service reform, tracing its conceptual and rhetorical roots as public management practice diverged from traditional public administration, took hold during the NPM reforms of the late 20th century, and evolved into more elaborate models of outcome-based management such as impact investment, outcomes funds, and social impact bonds in the recent 'governance' era.

We show how this evolution embodies an RTOC which combines the technical rationalism of management control systems theory (Kaplan and Norton 2015; Smith and Bititci 2017), with the behavioural rationalism of Public Choice Theory (Buchanan and Tulloch 1962) and Agency Theory (Jensen and Meckling 1976). By reviewing empirical evidence of the main instantiations of the RTOC, we find Pope Francis' stated reservations (Benedict XVI 2015) well justified: RTOC-derived approaches seem to deliver worse outcomes at greater cost.

The outcomes imperative in public service reform

Outcomes – defined in the broadest sense as indicators of societal wellbeing – have been an important policy consideration since at least the late 18th century. The Scottish Enlightenment figure John Sinclair (who popularised the term 'statistics') oversaw the *Statistical Account of Scotland* in 1791, the first nationwide account of social, economic, and agricultural conditions. Prior to this, national statistical accounts had 'uniformly been instituted, with a view of ascertaining the state of the country, for the purposes of taxation and war, and not of national improvement' (Sinclair 1798, p xxxv). Sinclair's intention, in line with the empiricist philosophy underpinning the Enlightenment, was to ascertain 'the quantum of happiness enjoyed by its inhabitants' (Sinclair 1798, p xiii) and guide national efforts for social improvement.

This ambition was taken up notably by the Statistical Societies established in major English and Welsh cities across the 1830s. The Manchester and London Statistical Societies – the only two still extant – both began statistical analysis of aggregate measures of social problems including crime, disease, and urban squalor. Social statistics became 'the "empirical arm" of political economy' (Porter 1986, p 27).

Over the course of the 20th century the measurement of outcomes expanded significantly with the development of post-war international organisations, in particular the United Nations (UN) and the Organization for Economic Cooperation and Development (OECD). The UN's Human Development Reports introduced in 1990 aimed to 'to shift the focus of development economics from national income accounting to people-centred policies'. The OECD's Better Life Index, established following the 2009 Stiglitz-Sen-Fitoussi Commission, helped spur a growing movement to reorientate focus from Gross Domestic Product to societal wellbeing. Perhaps the best known outcomes framework of all, the UN's 17 Sustainable Development Goals, describe a collective vision of global progress which is recognised by a majority of the world's population.

Few today would disagree that better measurement of societal outcomes can drive a more enlightened approach to statecraft. Given the significance of an outcomes agenda in public policy however, it is notable that no comparable influence was exerted on the development of *public administration* – the discipline concerning the resourcing and mobilisation of the machinery of governance – for much of the 20th century.

The development of the UK's post-war welfare state created large politically-controlled public bureaucracies, each focussed on broad social outcomes. The 'five giants' of want, disease, ignorance, squalor, and idleness, which underpinned the creation of Britain's modern welfare state, remain central themes of the social indicators monitored by many governments. The organisation and management of public services in the post-war period conformed to Max Weber's idea of a 'perfect bureaucracy', which could uphold values of universalism and fairness in the administration of public goods. Often called 'traditional' or 'bureaucratic' public administration, public administration during this time was strongly influenced by mechanistic approaches to management, such as Supply Chain Management, to organise activity through hierarchy and reductionism. While outcomes functioned as background indicators of social progress, they played a limited role in day-to-day activity since, 'high level goals provide little guide for action' (Simon 1957, p xxxvi).

Outcomes and new public management

Criticism of 'bureaucratic' public administration emerged from proponents of what came to be known as the NPM. NPM's intellectual heritage was strongly influenced by the laissez-faire Austrian School of economics which asserted the centrality of economic self-interest to social progress, and Public Choice Theory which extended the same assumptions to the public realm (Buchanan and Tulloch 1962). In this view, lacking any incentive for efficiency or customer satisfaction, public service officials could exploit their information-rich positions for self-gain at the expense of the public. A customer-oriented narrative was taken on by consultants and governments – citizens were 'frustrated with slow, unresponsive, inefficient bureaucracies that soak up ever more tax dollars and deliver ever poorer services' (Osborne and Gaebler 1992). Worse still, according to those authors, was the failure of traditional public administration to incentivise success: 'schools, welfare departments, and police departments typically get more money when they fail: when children do poorly, welfare roles swell, or the crime rate rises'.

NPM was mobilised by free market think tanks as the administrative arm of neoliberalism (James 1993). NPM advocated privatising state-owned organisations, breaking up public bodies into smaller and more specialised agencies, and introducing competition and quasi-markets into public service sectors. Where privatisation or marketisation were not possible for pragmatic or political reasons, the solution was to attach performance incentives, like target-linked payments, bonuses or reputational damage through naming and shaming, to the demonstration of results achieved. This would not just remedy traditional public administration's theorised deficiencies, but manifest an array of conceptual benefits including better-motivated employees, more innovative and entrepreneurial managers, improved transparency, and more direct public accountability (Bevan and Hood 2006; Heinrich 2002; Hood 1991).

In the UK, the Citizen's Charter introduced under John Major's Prime Ministership sought to guarantee a standard of customer responsiveness across sectors. The United States' Government Performance and Results Act of 1993 required federal agencies to conduct an annual regime of performance planning and reporting, the most high-profile example of a governmental push to 'work better and cost less' (Gore 1993). NPM created a new bargain for public managers: freedom from top-down performance controls in return for demonstrable success. In a speech following New Labour's election in 1997, UK Prime Minister Tony Blair announced his intention to lead 'a government that focuses on the outcomes it wants to achieve, devolves responsibility to those who can achieve those outcomes and then intervenes in inverse proportion to success' (Blair 1998, p 63). However, the results-based reforms subsequently imposed on public services – 'STAR' ratings for hospital managers, league tables for schools, and other public services and quasi-markets regulated by the UK state such as the energy and water utilities – operated in practice through using 'targets and terror' to coerce change from fearful public managers (Bevan and Hood 2006).

Early NPM reforms, for convenience, tended to focus on outputs rather than genuine outcomes; however, they became progressively outcome-oriented across the 1990s and early 2000s. The UK's 1998–2010 Public Service Agreements used to manage local government, for instance, steadily increased its proportion of outcome indicators relative to output targets with each of its iterations (Panchamia and Thomas 2014). As NPM's reach deepened in the Anglosphere and spread to other countries (see for example Borgonovi et al 2018), outcomes, which had previously functioned only as background indicators, became a central driver of service reform.

Outcomes and governance

While an outcomes orientation pulled towards a flexible, multi-agency operating basis, NPM was delivering the opposite. The advancement of NPM reforms transformed a centralised state into a fragmented and diminished entity dependent on networks and external organisations to accomplish the key tasks of governance. Privatisation, marketisation, and contracting out services to subsidiary agencies or external organisations progressively 'hollowed out' the state. The decentralisation and stratification of public services created new principal-agent divides between regulators and delivery organisations, funders and funding recipients, commissioners and contracted organisations, and among different tiers of government. This contributed to a layering of functions and more complex accountability relationships.

Accordingly, public administrations began a slow and partial transition from an NPM agenda towards one of 'governance' in the late nineties (Rhodes 1997). Taken broadly, governance constituted a different modality of state operation, not coercing or inducing through payment, but steering governance and policy networks, and working in various modalities of collaboration with a variety of external organisations. Governance was in many ways the natural administrative context for genuine outcome measures, whose determinants always lay beyond the organisational boundary.

A more recent concept attempting to bridge from NPM to a future pluralist governance landscape is 'New Public Governance' (Osborne 2010). Osborne proposed this model as a successor to NPM with its emphasis on inter-organisational working in a 'plural and pluralist' state. In practice, the outcome-based methods which were a core feature of NPM have not just survived this transition, but thrived.

In contemporary debates, outcomes are re-purposed as a governance logic, helping to steer and coordinate service systems fragmented and hollowed out by successive NPM reforms. Forms of outcome-based contracting like payment-by-results – in which payment is rendered for outcomes achieved not services rendered – had only a marginal role under early NPM but expanded significantly in the new millennium. The UK government's Open Public Services white paper in 2011 committed outcomes-based contracting to a central pillar of its service reform strategy. Flagship policy programmes like the Troubled Families Programme and Work Programme were designed on a payment-by-results basis (Crossley 2018), while payment-by-results contracting deepened in the administration of state international development aid.

Reconciling outcomes with a new governance context has required the innovation, not just expansion, of NPM methods. The most significant development has been the advancement of models of outcomes-based contracting and social investment, most clearly demonstrated by the growth and development of social impact bonds (SIBs). SIBs are forms of outcome-based contracting which broker private investment into social intervention, promising a rate of return based on outcomes achieved. SIBs offer a unique value proposition in a governance context: the ability to steer multiple parties within a contractual agreement, while transferring the risk of failure from resource-poor state commissioners to external investors. A second innovation, outcomes funds, are a mechanism whereby multiple funders pool together finance into a single funding stream to increase their incentive power and tackle higher-level and longer-term outcomes. By marshalling the contributions of numerous (potentially interlinked) outcome-based interventions, outcomes funds could achieve systemic effects beyond the domain of any one contractee.

Where NPM was advocated most notably by free market think tanks, SIBs, outcomes funds, and other outcome-based contracting mechanisms have been advocated by a broad assortment of philanthropic organisations, governments, and advisory groups. The number of SIBs has grown steadily over time since their introduction in the UK in 2007, spreading through the NPM heartland countries like the USA and Australia, and more recently advancing into many different countries where NPM was less influential. The Brookings Institution estimates by March 2022, 225 impact bonds had been established across 37 countries, totalling close to half a billion dollars in investment.

The Rationalist Theory of Outcome Creation

We have shown how a focus on outcomes has entrenched and persisted through the eras of traditional public administration, NPM, and into the era of governance. For NPM, outcome-based management promised to discipline indolent staff, prioritise customer value and free entrepreneurial public managers stifled by bureaucracy. In an era of governance, outcome-based management has been repackaged as a solution to the very problems it helped create, promising to help steer fragmented and hollowed-out public agencies while minimising the risk of innovation.

Common across all three phases of public administration has been an underlying model of improvement, wherein outcomes are achieved through a linear causal logic, production process, or value chain which link inputs to outcomes. This 'implicit model of the production process in the public sector' (Boyne and Law 2005, p 253) reflects a rationalist model of service production whereby inputs are structured into outputs through logical pathways which model processes in public services (for example, Pollitt and Bouckaert 2017). These outputs then interact with their environment and impact upon outcomes, following the simplified logic model adapted from Schedler and Proeller (2010) in Figure 2.1.

This model has a crucial operational significance. Outcomes are distinct from outputs in that they exist beyond organisational boundaries, yet in this perspective, they retain a deterministic link to preceding elements of the production chain. Building from French (2017), we term this an RTOC, which combines

Figure 2.1: The Rationalist Theory of Outcome Creation

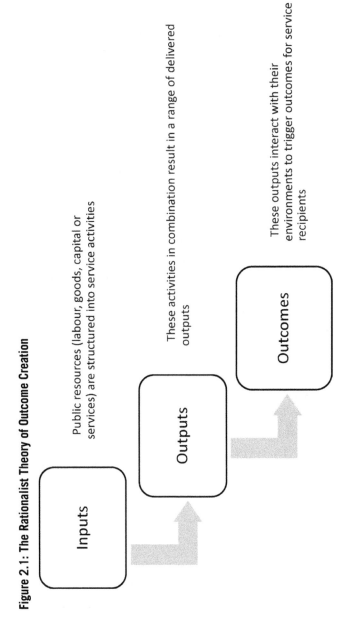

Public resources (labour, goods, capital or services) are structured into service activities

Inputs

These activities in combination result in a range of delivered outputs

Outputs

These outputs interact with their environments to trigger outcomes for service recipients

Outcomes

two core beliefs: a *technocratic* rationalism that the causes driving outcomes can be separated into component elements and impact assigned to individual contributions, with an *economic* rationalism that public servants are self-interested utility-maximisers whose behaviour can be predicted and controlled with extrinsic performance incentives. We briefly describe each position as follows.

Economic rationalism

The introduction of results-based reforms in the context of late NPM was motivated strongly by Public Choice Theory, which contended a fundamental divergence of interest between public officials and the populations they served. In this logic, lacking a market incentive analogous to commercial sector counterparts, public officials held little incentive to act in the public interest or to commit to improve their performance. Where behaviour was not regulated or intensively scrutinised, the autonomy of public managers would create 'agency costs', such as shirking or subversion.

The solution was to align public and private interests through coupling extrinsic performance incentives (payment or sanctions) on the demonstration of 'results' set by overseers, or 'principals' in Agency Theory terms (Jensen and Meckling 1976). In this way, self-interest could be harnessed as a productive motivational force and the coordination of staff or subsidiary units of organisation could be achieved through the design of incentive systems. Conditioning economic incentives on performance indicators and targets would align the incentives of all actors concerned – customers, staff, managers, and political overseers.

Technocratic rationalism

The utility of outcomes as a tool for accountability, improvement, and marketisation of public services depends on their objective measurement and the assessment of deterministic relationships between intra-organisational inputs and activities with outcomes. The model of outcome creation visualised in Figure 2.1 reflects the reductionist approach advocated by Herbert Simon in his *The Sciences of the Artificial* in which large problems are rendered manageable by decomposition into more legible and actionable sub-problems. It also reflects a rationalist philosophical belief of a Newtonian 'clockwork' universe in which social phenomena are driven by verifiable and immutable natural laws, and a Descartian 'systematic inquiry' in which the whole is examined through analysis of its parts.

In a public administration context, this underpinned Herbert Simon's dichotomy between a politicised policy process and a value-neutral administrative state. Writing about education, Smyth and Dow (1998, p 291) summarise the result of this: a drive to 'technologise schools, teaching and learning' and free decision making from 'the reliance on the teacher's value-laden, unreliable and subjective assessments' (Smyth and Dow 1998, p 298). Through adopting scientific measurement and evaluation methods, outcomes could be used to objectively account for the effectiveness of policies, public services, and social programmes, and hold those involved to account for their contribution.

The Rationalist Theory: fit for a complex world?

Instantiations of the RTOC promised two key benefits. First, the RTOC would create an improved incentive structure which aligns the divergent interests of service commissioners, employees, and users around the achievement of publicly-valued outcomes, motivating all parties to 'row' in the same direction. Shifting incentives from process compliance towards results achieved could spur innovative and entrepreneurial behaviour. Second, it would centre strategic decisions and assessments of attribution of performance upon a dispassionate assessment of objective performance information. Outcomes promised to set social interventions on an objective basis – helping winnow initiatives that work from those that don't and, through outcome-based contracts, paying for outcomes 'achieved' rather than services delivered. Whether one was a parent choosing the school in which to enrol their children, a school headteacher seeking to improve educational attainment, or a senior government official seeking to reform education policy, outcome-based management would create value through rational decision making.

Empirical evidence for both claims has been weak – and often contradictory – despite widespread interest and uptake of RTOC-derived models in many sectors and countries (Perrin 2007). A consistent finding is the difficulty of reconciling the elegant simplicity assumed by the RTOC with the complexity of its operating environments. Academic assessments of results-based management note intractable difficulties in measurement and attribution (Perrin 2007; Wimbush 2011; Bovaird 2014; Jamieson et al 2020). More troublingly, the literature also documents a range of performance paradoxes, wherein its implementation has actually undermined performance (van Thiel and Leeuw 2002; Bevan and Hood 2006; Lowe and Wilson 2017). While a comprehensive review of these problems is beyond the scope of this book, we take stock of four key recurring problems.

The measurement problem

The RTOC takes as given that outcomes can be represented as objective, standardised quantitative indicators. Cartwright et al (2016) argue that while some outcomes can be measured as 'pinpoint' concepts (relatively precise and unambiguous measures like mortality or disease incidence), many others like family, poverty, disability, or health are multi-faceted, contested, and subjective concepts. The authors term these

'Ballung' concepts which serve multiple valid interpretations and reconstructions, and can only be represented subjectively by proxy indicators. The authors note that even fundamental concepts like 'health' and 'disease' have resisted reduction to pinpoint criteria. Outcome measures in the social domain – wellbeing, social cohesion, level of education – are even further from consensus, with key dimensions evolving in concert with shifting social attitudes. 'Ballung' outcome measures are always imperfect, since single measures can only capture (and therefore privilege) one aspect of a multidimensional problem or human experience, while indices or weighted 'baskets' of indicators introduce subjectivity and arbitrariness into indicator design. Crucially, both routes compromise the objectivity upon which rational decision making depends.

Measurement problems also influence operational capability of outcomes-based management systems. The demand of the RTOC for objective, unified, quantitative indicators can easily skew focus towards more straightforwardly or more inexpensively measured elements, while those outcomes and indicators more difficult to reconcile become sidelined (Wilson et al 2011). This can lead to the well-documented phenomena whereby 'what's measured is what matters' (Bevan and Hood 2006; Lowe and Wilson 2017), and where targets are assigned, to 'hitting the target but missing the point'.

The attribution problem

The RTOC necessitates the determination of attribution to movement in indicators and assumes a deterministic link between activities and outcomes. This depends critically on the ability to attribute movement in measured indicators to prior actions. In practice there is often an unclear direction of travel from organisational outputs to societal outcomes, which can depend on many intermediate steps, each of which may be uncertain or be poorly evidenced. Unlike outputs, outcomes are dynamically impacted by a range of unpredictable and uncontrollable external factors which resist disaggregation to the inputs of any particular organisation, initiative, or activity (Bovaird 2014; Cornford et al 2013).

Even factors which do improve outcomes may involve significant time lags in determining impact, stretching beyond funding terms and even political cycles. Outcomes are determined not by the positive impact of interventions – for example increased police activities reducing measured crime rates – but through tackling upstream factors and preventing negative outcomes – for instance criminal recidivism – from emerging. Achieving such 'maintenance outcomes' can take many years to materialise and require expensive and limiting control group evaluations to assess.

The incentive problem

Performance incentives have proved extremely effective motivators of organisational behaviour – but not of the intended form. Actors cannot reasonably be held to account over factors which contribute to outcomes but lie beyond their control. Where strong performance incentives are imposed regardless, incentives are created to manipulate the factors of practice which are under control: changing behaviour to focus on measured elements rather than value-creating activity (Bevan and Hood 2006), or skewing, distorting, or forging performance information (van Thiel and Leeuw 2002). To take just one example, the UK government's Troubled Families Programme claimed a 99 per cent rate of success in 'turning around' family problems, until an evaluation showed that councils were gaming the system by intervening only in those cases where families were guaranteed to reach target criteria (see Crossley 2018). This is far from an isolated case – a systematic review of evidence of target-based performance management reported that 81 per cent of studies reviewed indicated gaming behaviour, the same proportion found altered social relationships, and 74 per cent found evidence of outright falsification (Franco-Santos and Otley 2018).

Both Campbell's Law and Goodhart's Law explain that performance targets always create perverse incentives. Using outcomes as targets amplifies this problem because they lie beyond the ability of any individual agent to bring about independently or predictably. Those subject to performance management regimes therefore face a significant incentive to take shortcuts – by skewing, withholding, distorting, or forging performance data. This creates an intractable problem for RTOC-derived approaches: they cannot use performance data to make people accountable without corrupting the measurement and attribution processes on which they rely.

The control problem

The problems discussed so far relate to limitations in gathering together the knowledge to measure outcomes, evaluate interventions, or monitor whether productive or perverse behaviour is undertaken by performance-managed staff. However, even if it were possible to remedy all of these factors, there would still be the substantial problem of mounting an effective systemic response to match the scale and complexity of target outcomes. Through its reliance on prediction and control, the RTOC presumes the existence of a sufficiently powerful authority able to assign and enforce accountabilities and mete out rewards or sanctions. However the fragmentation of public service landscapes and layering of accountabilities – itself partly facilitated by outcomes-based methods – have increasingly necessitated collaboration and cooperation in governance networks (Christensen and Lægreid 2007).

Assessing the feasibility of the Rationalist Theory of Outcome Creation

Responses to the challenges discussed have fallen into two camps. The first has treated these issues as technical challenges to be reconciled by more sophisticated (yet paradigmatically consistent) strategies, tools, and models. Boyne and Law (2005) for instance claim the 'wicked issues' of outcome-based management can be addressed through better outcome indicator design and more strategic planning. Heinrich (2002) similarly advises paying close attention to choosing indicators which are well-aligned with outcomes, which are inexpensive to administer, and which make it difficult to improve through means other than improving performance directly. Pollitt et al (2010) argue that indicator and incentive systems should be regularly refreshed to shake off the gaming routines which have embedded.

More strident critics would contend that this reconciliatory approach is an attempt to square the circle. Lowe and Wilson (2017) for instance assert that results-based management gamify services themselves, and therefore will *always* encourage gaming behaviour. Miller (2014) writes similarly how the managerial 'proving' agenda behind outcomes will *always* subvert and distort their 'improving' potential. For Smyth and Dow (1998, p 291), outcomes 'promise of a semblance of order, control, and certainty', but *always* deliver the opposite, while for Soss et al (2011), gaming results not from aberrations or misapplications of RTOC models and methods, but 'predictable products of core contradictions'. Many are reaching the same conclusion: *the simplicity demanded by the RTOC is fundamentally incompatible with the complexity of the real world.*

Summary

Our conclusion is that the evident limitations to the RTOC, taken together, signify a paradigmatic crisis (Kuhn 1962). It is the innate and intractable complexity of outcomes – their immeasurability, externality, ambiguity, and causal uncertainty – which undermines the RTOC as a meaningful architecture for outcomes improvement in all but the most simplistic and exceptional of situations. We argue that only a deeper and more realistic conceptual understanding of how outcomes are created – or indeed emerge – can provide a way forward.

THREE

The Complexity Theory
of Outcome Creation

Writing more than two decades ago, Smyth and Dow (1998, p 291) wrote that 'outcomes appear to have become part of a naturalised and largely uncontested discourse', which has 'rendered others irrelevant'. Recently however, public management scholarship has begun to engage seriously with the measurement and management of social outcomes as a theoretical and conceptual matter. A viable and compelling alternative conception to the RTOC has since developed within public health, social epidemiology and health geography scholarship, positioning outcomes not as products of service production chains, but as the emergent properties of complex systems. We expand on this model in a public administration context to construct an alternative model, the CTOC.

Outcomes as emergent properties of complex systems

From a sociological perspective, it has been long understood that social outcomes are systemic problems, not programmatic results. Published in 1897, Emile Durkheim's *Suicide: A Study in Sociology* contended population-level suicide rates were an irreducible product of social structure, explained by the dynamic interaction between individual psychological factors and social norms. Social epidemiologists more recently have argued that complex social structures create distributions of population health. In the UK, the Black Report found significant associations between widening health inequalities and other key outcomes, particularly discrepancies in economic opportunity (Department of Health and Social Security 1980). The World Health Organization's Commission on the Social Determinants of Health linked health inequalities to a much wider array of factors such as governance quality, social policy, social norms, and wider economic trends (WHO 2008), and a more recent review by the Health Foundation found only 10 per cent of population health was related to access to quality health care.

Action to address the 'social determinants of health' has been a growing focus of the public health community, with a consistent recommendation to refocus from reactive spending to tackling the latent causes responsible for structuring patterns of unequal outcomes (Marmot and Wilkinson 2005). Rather than searching for single 'upstream' factors as root causes for poor or unequal outcomes coupled with an associated set of interventions targeted at individual change, Schensul (2009) argued that it was the interaction of factors across multiple areas which explained emergent distributions of outcomes.

Theorists from disciplines of public health, social epidemiology, and health geography have drawn from the systems and complexity sciences to engage constructively with the systemic implications of health outcomes (Gattrell 2005; Curtis and Riva 2010; Finegood 2011; Jayasinghe 2011, 2015; Carey et al 2015; Fink et al 2016; Gatzweller et al 2017; Rutter et al 2017). Jayasinghe (2011, p 1), for instance, argued we should understand 'population health outcomes as an emergent property of (Complex Adaptive Systems), which has numerous dynamic non-linear interactions among its interconnected sub-systems or agents', while Fink et al (2016, p 98) contended

Figure 3.1: The UK Government Office for Science Obesity Systems Map

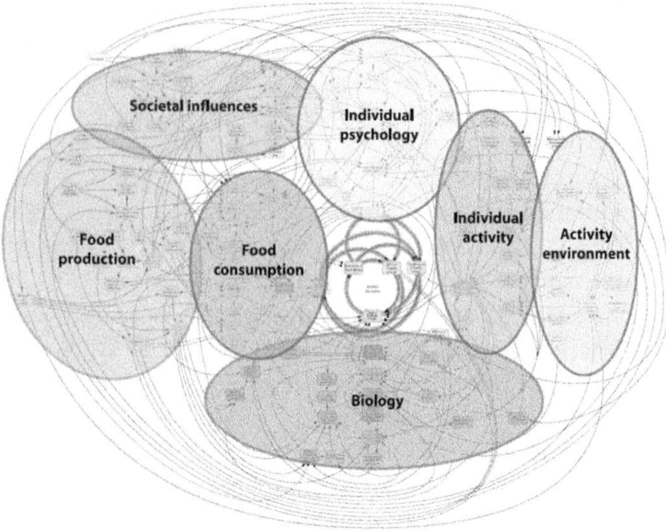

Source: Adapted from Vandenbroeck et al 2007

all health outcomes 'emerge from the complex interplay of health-related factors at multiple levels, from the biological to the societal level'.

This view offers a fundamentally different conception of outcomes to the RTOC perspective, because outcomes are shaped by interdependent, dynamically interacting factors far beyond the individual or organisational boundary that cannot be wholly separated into component parts. As an illustrative example, Figure 3.1 presents the findings of a 2007 attempt to 'look under the hood' of obesity by using a causal loop diagram to model the interconnected and nested sets of factors spanning psychological, social, economic, and environmental spheres (Vandenbroeck et al 2007).

The obesity map provides a stark visual counterpoint to the 'rationalist' logic visualised in Figure 2.1 in the previous chapter. Obesity is shown in the centre of the diagram, emerging from the dynamic interaction of a constellation of factors spanning multiple nested systems, including individual, biological, and psychological processes, and broader systemic factors like food production systems and social norms around healthy eating. The map's authors hoped that by facilitating an attention to system dynamics the obesity map would lead to actionable insight and guide policy design and the strategic positioning of interventions. In this ambition, however, the map has been a failure. Policymakers who might have sought greater understanding and guidance for leveraging investments or designing new legislation found themselves instead paralysed by the sheer scale and messiness of complexity. Indeed, its lack of actionability has landed the map with the epithet 'horrendogram' in the public health community.

But what if the real value of the map was not to inform but to confound its audience – drawing attention to the problem rather than the solution? In this section, we undertake a deeper exploration of the four dimensions of complexity which characterise the emergence of outcomes, only one of which is recognised in the obesity map and much public health scholarship. By better appreciating the complexity of outcome creation across all four dimensions, we argue greater actionable insight can be achieved.

Compositional complexity

The first dimension of complexity is the only form captured by the obesity diagram. 'Compositional complexity' refers to the multiplicity, interdependency, and diversity of component factors, whose interrelationships collectively determine outcomes at any given point. Complexity theory cautions us that constituent elements of complex systems are causally interdependent and mutually reinforcing, and therefore that causal products are emergent phenomena; that is, they are higher-order factors which are irreducible to individual constituent factors. The obesity map shows the presence of strong feedback loops arising from the densely interconnected nature of factors within overlapping and nested systems. These sustain emergent outcomes and resist external shocks: isolated interventions operating on just one or a small number of areas are unlikely to achieve systemic impact (Finegood et al 2011).

Compositional complexity is underpinned by the key features of multiplicity and diversity of component parts, and by interdependency, frequency of interaction, and feedback loops defining how factors interrelate to produce emergent outcomes. The implication here is that any reasonable measure of performance is based not on the efficiency of individual elements but by their interrelationships (Melnyk et al 2014; Bourne et al 2018). Thus, health outcomes lie beyond the ability of primary healthcare services to resolve alone, educational outcomes transcend the ability of schools to achieve independently, and crime and recidivism outcomes lie beyond the jurisdiction of the police and criminal justice organisations. Compositional complexity therefore serves to stop people thinking principally in terms of the effectiveness of individual organisations or interventions, and more about how to meaningfully engage with the systems they are embedded within. The core message of the Foresight Programme which introduced the obesity map was, 'the need for broad and diversified policies or strategies to change the dynamics of the system' (Vandenbroeck et al 2007, p 8).

Experiential complexity

Compositional complexity is acknowledged in public health scholarship in the dynamics of a unified, aggregate model of population outcomes, in effect obscuring important qualitative differences in how outcomes are determined and experienced across populations. While outcomes are modelled at the population level, the conditions which lead any particular individual into and out of key outcome states like obesity, homelessness, or poverty are highly individuated, and the range of appropriate responses ought to be similarly varied to be effective. Experiential complexity refers to the variety of experience in how outcomes are achieved and how they are valued and prioritised in different people's lives.

The obesity diagram consists of 108 factors which are held to collectively determine aggregate population-level dynamics. While many of these can only be tackled through high-level political agendas, new legislation and regulation of the food production industry, a large proportion of others, particularly individual, psychological and biological components, are understood to vary from individual to individual. Modelling outcomes at a population level therefore abstracts a stylised picture of a highly individuated process, with variable accuracy. In fact, by aggregating and generalising constitutive factors, resulting models may not adequately depict *any* individual experience. While population-level modelling promises greater mastery of complexity, to fully map out a national outcome like obesity we would require a separate (though interconnected) obesity diagram for every individual in the country.

Coping with experiential complexity requires engaging with Ashby's (1956) Law of Requisite Variety: viable systems require the ability to at least match the variety of demand presented by their operating environment. While private businesses can choose to target specific cohorts of customers, public organisations must respond to a great diversity of lived experience among the citizenry, often with urgent, multiple, and intersecting needs and capabilities. By reducing outcomes to unified proxy indicators, or aggregating experiences into broad causal factors, we strip away the experiential dynamics of outcome creation. This is problematic since outcomes can only be co-produced with the consent, support, and expertise of the individuals experiencing them. At times, the values and beliefs which shape how core societal outcomes are created – for instance justice, democracy, or wellbeing – may create resistance to a single universalising conception of outcomes and endangers 'producing an approximately right solution to the wrong problem' (Dunn 2017, p 73). For instance, New Zealand's Living Standards Framework, a holistic, societal-level measurement system to assess population wellbeing, presented a Westernised view of collective wellbeing and had to be reimagined through an indigenous interpretation (the *He Ara Waiora*) based on alternative values of communitarianism and self-determination.

Dynamic complexity

The dimensions of complexity discussed so far give the impression of a static and closed system, bound together through stable configurations of causal factors. In reality, the constituent factors which determine outcome emergence are in a constant state of flux and disequilibrium. Dynamic complexity refers to the churn and volatility of causal factors and their interrelationships through which outcomes emerge.

Uncontrollable and often unpredictable changes in economic conditions, technological advancement, environmental change, and social attitudes set the environment in which policies, services, and social interventions operate. Outcomes are created in open systems which challenge the enduring relevance of services and social interventions in an evolving performance landscape.

The more visible source of dynamic complexity may be large system-changing shocks which impact whole populations. The COVID-19 pandemic and associated policy change is the obvious recent example, however at the individual level similarly significant shocks happen far more readily. Employment termination, relationship breakdowns, or sudden homelessness, can be similarly impactful and system changing.

Representations of causal factors, for example through system mapping, face an obvious threat to their enduring relevance. The obesity map is a snapshot of system dynamics, and much will has changed in the years since it was produced. Causal models, simulations, and predictions based on causal composition run the risk of losing relevance and utility and wasting the effort involved in their construction, or worse still, misleading their audiences by omitting significant changes. The systems used to control and regulate organisations are also challenged – strategic plans may lose expediency, while control-oriented performance management systems cannot assist managerial processes 'without constraining the speed of decision making and action that we now need to be successful' (Melnyk et al 2014, p 179).

Dynamic complexity means that evidence-based policies and social interventions have a half-life: their effectiveness decays over time decay as conditions evolve. The capacity to adapt, that is, to make sense of changes and respond to new operating contexts, rather than effectiveness and efficiency, becomes the central design principle. This would mean the ability to reformulate strategy, organisational functions, and management approaches to accommodate changes affecting multiple levels of outcome systems, from the micro (individual level) to the meso (for example community-level or organisational level) to the macro (for example policy change, economic, social and cultural shifts).

Governance complexity

Compositional, experiential, and dynamic complexities, taken together, create key epistemic limitations to pursuing outcomes. Any actor – be they policymakers, public service professionals, or individuals experiencing particular outcome states – are challenged by fundamental limitations to their ability to predict or hold certainty about means-ends relationships. However, even if sufficient knowledge were possessed, another challenge would remain in mobilising a coordinated systemic response of suitable scale to tackle target outcomes effectively. Governance complexity therefore refers to the task of mobilising and coordinating the diverse knowledges, relationships, and resources over the long time periods necessary to impact on outcomes.

Outcomes are invariably trans-boundary in nature, and ordinarily lie across institutional remits and accountabilities. Even in situations of strong alignment, for example the association of educational attainment with schools, the overall contribution of exogenous factors may prove more significant than the value provided from service provision. Outcomes inevitably spill out of ring-fenced budgets, transcend organisational boundaries, and operate across cultural divisions among different organisations and service sectors. As public service landscapes have fragmented and decentralised through successive NPM reforms, accountability relationships have layered and complexified with no single actor in complete control.

Public service systems with which citizens interact therefore have increasingly themselves resembled complex systems, characterised by multiple interacting, self-organising, and semi-autonomous agents with power and influence dispersed across the relationships among them (Eppel and Rhodes 2018; Uhl-Bien et al 2007). This brings into focus the practice of governance in which forms of steering, collaboration, integration, and co-creation take precedence over control and competition.

A general complexity perspective on outcome creation

Despite the obesity map's visual complexity, it captures only one dimension – compositional complexity. Dynamic complexity explains that the map is a snapshot of system dynamics, much of which have changed over the years since it was produced. It is also an abstracted and aggregated picture which ignores the innate experiential complexity through which outcomes are achieved, prioritised, and valued across populations. Governance complexity is overlooked by the map's emphasis on policymakers as its key audience.

Public health scholarship has in general derived from a particular philosophical tradition in the complexity sciences allied with what Edgar Morin (2006) described as a 'restricted' model of complexity. The close association between many studies and a 'complex adaptive systems' model, the flagship intellectual contribution of the Santa Fe Institute, typifies this affiliation. In this literature, policy architects are directed to identify the key 'leverage points' where targeted action may lead to system-changing effects. Indeed, the methods which predominate in the policy literature to cope with complexity – for example models of system description (such as systems dynamics or causal loop modelling) or simulation (such as agent-based modelling) hold as their core purpose the attempt to wrestle complexity into a manageable format, with complexity functioning as Edgar Morin described 'as a kind of wagon behind the truth locomotive' (Morin 2006, p 6). Complexity is positioned as policy superpower, permitting mastery over a class of problems which have long proven resistant to the standard policy toolkit. The prescription is to deal with complexity through an additional step in the policy cycle. The result is a further affirmation of the power of governments, funders, and senior managers of social interventions to deliver outcomes at scale.

Our depiction of a dynamic, individualised, and causally complex outcome creation process spanning multiple system scales process sits at odds with this 'restricted' understanding, conforming instead to a 'general' complexity worldview, to use Morin's (2006) and, later, Byrne and Callaghan's (2014) language. In this perspective, human intentions cannot be reduced to reliable and codifiable behavioural characteristics, and the interaction of dissimilar actors across multiple scales leads to an unpredictable and irreducible form of emergence. This takes place amid a dynamic environment over which any agent has little control and, likely, limited knowledge of forthcoming events. General complexity initiates not merely a methodological departure from rationalism, but a fundamental epistemological rethinking which Morin describes as paradigmatic.

The modelling of relationships between system 'wholes' and component parts will necessarily involve subjective interpretations, constrained by the standpoint of any given individual within a system. It is not possible for a single actor, however central, to possess complete knowledge of the system – and after a point of specificity, counterproductive to try. The patterns of emergence determining outcomes instead conforms to a 'complex realism' viewpoint which assumes a real but unknowable and unforecastable systemic composition (Byrne and Callaghan 2014). The outcome creation process resembles less the static diagram of the obesity model, and more a non-repeating pattern of unpredictable individual components. As discussed in the introduction, we prefer the visual analogy of Penrose tiling to the obesity map – public service follows an unpredictable, dynamically unfolding pattern, in which key decisions made (to follow the Penrose analogy, whether to attach a kite or rhombus shape to the pattern) shape the future in significant and unpredictable ways.

Summary: contrasting theories of outcome creation

In this chapter we have described the contours of what we contend is a novel alternative theoretical conception of how positive social outcomes are created and sustained. We call this a Complexity Theory of Outcome Creation, which we contend is structured across four dimensions:

- Compositional complexity, which results from the interdependence and inter-determinacy of causal systems from which outcomes emerge.
- Dynamic complexity, which results from the volatility and flux of interacting causal factors and their operating environment.
- Experiential complexity, which results from the variety of ways in which outcomes are experienced, prioritised and navigated by individuals.

- Governance complexity, which results from the distribution of knowledge, agency, and resources needed to tackle outcomes across a range of independent actors.

The complexity of outcomes cannot be treated, as public health and public policy scholarship has largely contended, as a policy issue for governments, policymakers, funders, and senior managers. Instead, the requisite knowledge and capabilities to address outcomes are spread across a fragmented and resource-poor administrative landscape – a situation exacerbated itself by the application of existing outcome-based management techniques. Building on the philosophical positions of Cilliers (2002), Morin (2006) and Byrne and Callaghan (2014), we extend the public health understanding of outcomes as emergent products of complex systems into a philosophical context of general complexity. Table 3.1 contrasts the core assumptions of both RTOC and CTOC.

The RTOC combines technocratic rationalism – a Newtonian view of a clockwork universe predicated on underlying causal certainty – with economic rationalism – that extrinsic incentives are best placed to coordinate a public sector workforce motivated by self-interest. The CTOC instead issues from Morin's general complexity worldview, wherein a 'strong' emergence derives from the largely unknowable interactions of a broad array of diverse factors, itself a property of the four forms of complexity inherent to outcomes. This means that the requisite knowledge and power needed to tackle outcomes effectively is spread across a large range of actors, many beyond the control of formal accountabilities and organisational hierarchies.

Instances of the RTOC have included management techniques like pay-for-success schemes, logframe project management, payment-by-results contracting, SIBs and outcome funds. In the next chapter we consider how our CTOC might provide a constructive basis for the design of social interventions, thus serving as an alternative catalyst for innovation in public service reform.

Table 3.1: Philosophical assumptions of the Rationalist and Complexity Theories of Outcome Creation

	Rationalist Theory of Outcome Creation (RTOC)	Complexity Theory of Outcome Creation (CTOC)
Conceptual understanding	Outcomes are the cumulative products of inputs, throughputs and outputs	Outcomes are emergent properties of complex systems
Improvement approach	Outcomes are improved through well-designed social interventions administered by extrinsically motivated employees	Outcomes are improved by meaningful engagement with four forms of complexity: compositional, dynamic, experiential, and governance
Causal claims	**Determinism.** Outcomes are real, measureable, and causation is determined by a set of natural laws – hierarchy, linearity, and reductionism. Social intervention is a closed system	**General complexity.** Outcomes are determined by open complex systems whose dynamics cannot be reduced to constituent parts. Causality is characterised by non-linearity, feedback loops, and instability
Knowledge claims	**Rationalism.** Theory and reason underpin universal assumptions about knowledge. Objective knowledge is privileged according to an evidence hierarchy epitomised by experiments and systematic reviews	**Humility.** Knowledge about outcomes is contested and context-specific. The experiential knowledge of citizens and frontline staff are crucial inputs alongside traditional scientific evidence
Theory of human behaviour	**Economic rationalism.** Behaviour is governed by self-interest, and can be mobilised towards outcomes through the extrinsic performance incentive systems	**Bounded rationality and optimism.** Systems are too complex to be knowable, and decisions must be taken in situations of considerable uncertainty. Intrinsic motivation and value-led cooperation may be the only possible means of behaviour change

FOUR

Complexity as a service reform trajectory: dynamic capabilities for better public service outcomes

The CTOC contends that the effectiveness of services and interventions is determined not by the efficiency of internal processes, but by how effectively public service systems can engage with the innate complexity of the systems from which outcomes emerge. In this chapter we transpose the challenges posed by complexity into design parameters for public service reform. We draw from Teece et al's (1997) theory of dynamic capabilities to articulate three core capabilities we consider necessary in tackling complex outcomes: stewardship, coordination, and adaptation. We argue that investment in and management of these three capabilities in consort could inform an alternative logic of outcome-focussed service reform.

Complexity as a public administration problem

Policymakers and policy analysts have shown increasing interest in complexity, though have tended to be drawn toward a 'restricted complexity' model, in which complexity is wrestled into the policy cycle through more adopting appropriate strategic tools and methodologies like systems mapping, computational simulations, or forecasting (see for example Barbrook-Johnson and Penn 2022).

In our theoretical perspective, complexity is foremost a problem for public *administration*, not public policy. The people best placed to create value are not policymakers or service leaders, but those at the core of service interaction – citizens and person-facing professionals – who are best capable of sensing and responding to the lived complexity of outcomes. While we think complexity-informed policy tools have an important role to play, they are secondary to addressing the distribution of agency in public services. Further, rather than 'tooling up' existing roles in policy processes (for example policy analyst, project manager, evaluator) with complexity-informed skills, altogether different roles may be needed (for example system convenor, network weaver, learning partner). Table 4.1 shows how complexity creates an imbalance of agency and information across the policy-administration divide.

The table shows how the four forms of complexity at the heart of the CTOC structure different problems across four key administrative roles. For practitioners, informational problems (for example how one individual varies from another, or how needs have changed over time) are keenly sensed. This group is constrained by their limited power to move beyond role boundaries, and often their obligations to follow standard operating procedures or hit preordained targets rather than work to create value for the people they work with. Those who currently have most agency – significantly, policymakers and service commissioners operating at a distance from practice – cannot access the information necessary to provide effective intervention. Instead, the requisite knowledge and capabilities to address outcomes are spread across a fragmented and resource-poor administrative landscape. The table illustrates a core dilemma: *our system of administering public services means those with the best ability to improve outcomes have the least agency to do so.*

Table 4.1: Outcome complexity as a public administration problem

High ◄——— Information ◄——— Low

Public Service Role	Compositional Complexity	Experiential Complexity	Dynamic Complexity	Governance Complexity
Frontline practitioner	The problems which I am confronted with are multi-faceted – it is not always clear where to start	The problems and capabilities of people I encounter vary widely, requiring very different approaches to achieve the best result	The problems and capabilities held by my service users are different today than they were last week, requiring a different strategy	I need rapid support from others with different expertise and resources to respond adequately
Service or project manager	The problems our target groups face require support beyond far beyond just single interventions	My service must tailor responses adequately to the individual context of each person who engages with us	My service must cope with different challenges and demands from those we were set up to address	My service must work in lockstep with other agencies and collaborators to achieve goals
Service commissioner	The populations I serve have deeply enmeshed needs, often requiring multiple interlinked interventions	The services I commission must respond to a wide range of potential needs and capabilities	Population needs are constantly evolving: the services I commission today may soon no longer fit their context	My service must work in lockstep with other agencies, who we may have no formal service agreements with, to achieve goals
Policymaker	Policies must be holistic and interconnected to tackle many different interacting problems, not just single issues	High-level policies lack relevance to individual contexts and directives can constrain the power of better-informed actors to adapt	Policies must be revised and updated based on an evolving understanding of problems	Policies can establish high-level institutional structures and procedures, but cannot provide relevant sufficient detail for action

Low ——————► Agency ——————► High

The necessity of professional agency in achieving policy goals is a central tenet of public administration scholarship, and perhaps best codified in Michael Lipsky's concept of 'street-level bureaucracy' (Lipsky 1971). In this view, policy success is determined by the discretion of those actors many stages downstream from policy development. Our position reaffirms this – public administration remains the missing link in ensuring public services and social interventions contribute meaningfully to population-level social outcomes.

Yet complexity has a reputation as a negative force which thwarts the best intentions of programme designers and public managers. In contrast, it is common to find complexity theory adopted as a constructive framework in organisational theory and business management, with links to innovation, creativity, and resilience (Boulton et al 2015; Jackson 2019). In the following section, and indeed the rest of this book, we apply complexity as a constructive design principle to approach public service reform.

Toward complexity-capable public services?

We have argued for a rebalancing of agency toward the relational core of public service interaction. In this section we build on this argument to consider how the capabilities necessary to engage with the dynamic, intractable, and variable nature of public service demand can be developed.

One way of approaching this problem is through the lens of what Professor David Teece has called 'dynamic capabilities'. An organisation's capabilities, Teece et al (1997) argued, could be static (that is embedded in established operational procedures), or dynamic (that is they renew operational capabilities in response to or in anticipation of changes in an external environment). The latter were described as an organisation's, 'ability to integrate, build and reconfigure internal and external competences to address rapidly changing environments' (Teece et al 1997, p 516). A similar concept in complexity theory is the idea of a system's 'adaptive capacity', its ability to sense and respond to environmental changes to ensure its organisational fitness.

While Teece's concept was developed in a context of profit-seeking private organisations, it has been used in a public sector context for understanding the reconfiguration and renewal of capabilities in public sector organisations (for example Pablo et al 2007; Piening 2013; Kattel and Mazzucato 2018). We use the term slightly differently, focussing instead on the capabilities demonstrated within public service *systems*, not merely organisations, to match the multi-level and trans-boundary nature of social outcomes. This extends from beyond the static capability of 'discretion' afforded to individual street-level bureaucrats in public administration scholarship (Lipsky 1971). Dynamic capabilities in this context are an appropriate concept to situate a practical focus on the process of constant reconfiguration necessitated by our conception of an outcome creation process which is dynamic, non-linear, multi-faceted, and individuated.

While the RTOC views outcomes as created through efficient services, competitive markets and well-designed policies, the CTOC assumes outcomes will be improved through investment in the requisite dynamic capabilities to govern the inherent complexity of outcome-oriented public service. In the next section we outline three capabilities which might serve as the core focal points behind such a complexity-relevant administrative praxis.

Stewardship capability

The epistemic limitations brought about by compositional, experiential, and dynamic complexities mean it is not possible to specify in detail the measures, actions, or operating procedures necessary to improve outcomes on a consistent basis. Instead, it is the creativity, resilience, and adaptability of public service professionals in navigating uncertainty, not their task efficiency, which is the engine of improvement. Attempts to constrain the agency of staff through coercive targets or operating procedures will instead demotivate and misdirect public service work.

Part of the problem is the continued attachment of management and accountability systems on the presumption of self-interest, with principal-agent relationships the core dynamic for structuring service delivery and contractual work (for example Heinrich 2002). An alternative relational basis can be derived from Davis et al's (1997) 'Stewardship Theory': assume that public service officials can be trusted to operate independently as stewards of the public good rather than agents of their own self-interest. While 'agents' will connive to shirk or misappropriate resources given the chance, stewards are driven by 'a shared sense of ongoing responsibility to multiple stakeholders, which affects a focus on collective welfare over the long term' (Hernandez 2012, p 176). The first requisite capability for dealing with complexity is therefore stewardship: the capability of public service professionals to act as responsible stewards of publicly-valued outcomes.

This perspective would approach service design and management from a position of trust rather than suspicion in the motivations and professionalism of the public service workforce, and presume alignment in the goals sought by staff and their organisation. The intrinsic and goal-directed motivation of stewards towards improvement fits well with the requirements for experimentation, sense-making, learning, and adaptation long recognised as necessary for improvement in complex environments (Kurtz and Snowden 2003). Where agents are controlled by specific targets and extrinsic incentive systems, stewards respond to values, principles, and role boundaries which are far more relevant and applicable to conditions which are uncertain, novel, or ambiguous. We consider that capability for stewardship provides an alternative motivational and behavioural basis for public management.

Such an optimistic viewpoint may be considered naïve, particularly when standards of accountability operate largely on 'agency theory' assumptions. Stewardship is an assumption most often reserved for those in leadership roles. In the UK, the 'good chap' convention entrusts political leaders to operate with integrity in the public interest in the absence of a codified constitutional settlement (Blick and Hennessey 2019). Those most capable of improving outcomes in public services, practitioner officers and frontline staff, are afforded no such courtesy, consigned to the bottom of organisational hierarchies and subjected in many instances to increasing regulation, cost pressure, and erosion of professional identities. The evidence contradicts this settlement. Workforce surveys have consistently found high levels of motivation toward the values of public service in public and non-profit services relative to private sector counterparts (Perry et al 2010), while much frontline policy work innately depends on value-motivated public service professionals (Lipsky 1971). Public trust in the political leaders who enjoy autonomy through the 'good chap' convention is meanwhile historically low, and in the UK has deteriorated further still over recent years (Heydecker et al 2022).

Second, stewardship is a capability not a presumption – it can be developed or confounded by the actions taken and decisions made by organisational leaders. Public service functions could be designed to support stewards and stewarding rather than to constrain agents. Capability for stewardship could become a core criteria of HR processes like recruitment, career progression, and performance reviews. Performance measurement systems could be established to work in service of those administering public services, rather than to coax efficiency gains from them through coercion. Proceeding from a basis of trust may also provide a rationale to reduce tiresome and bureaucratic reporting burdens, freeing service professionals to engage more fully in value-creating work (Romzek and Dubnick 1987). Leadership could be focussed on enabling environments rather than controlling behaviour (Mintzberg and Waters 1985), ensuring organisational procedures support and reward stewardship behaviours while accommodating risks this might involve (Heifetz et al 2009).

We see stewardship as a collaborative concept, operating across agencies and multiple levels of organisations (Hallsworth 2011). Stewardship – due to compositional and governance complexities – necessarily also extends beyond the organisational boundary. Organisational leaders can still embody stewardship by modelling expected behaviours and setting a permissive environment for the risky and emotionally-involved decision-making processes necessitated by effective stewardship. Those with significant budgetary authority including high-level managers, service commissioners, and planners need to take on a collective stewardship of outcomes and ensure this, rather than narrow organisational matters, remains the strategic focus (Lowe et al 2021b). Leaders can also embody stewardship by operating as system leaders and system thinkers, seeking impact beyond the operations of their organisations, and seeking to embolden a collective sense of stewardship beyond the organisational boundary (Hobbs 2019).

Coordinative capability

Stewardship capability provides a means to legitimise and promote an informed responsiveness to desired outcomes within and across organisations (Davis et al 1997). The cross-boundary, causally uncertain, and co-produced nature of outcomes requires the integration of resources, relationships, knowledge, and commitments from across professional and cultural boundaries (Rhodes 1997; Osborne 2010). Stewardship capability is therefore not by itself enough. Public service professionals must be able to access and actively integrate the collective intelligence and distributed resources across public service systems to mount any effective systemic response. We define this second necessary dynamic capability as 'coordinative capability': the ability to shape patterns of interaction to mobilise and interpret the requisite knowledge, resources, and procedures necessary to improve outcomes.

Coordinative capability requires actors to develop and act on a critical systemic awareness of the opportunities which may exist beyond their immediate organisational or role boundaries. The capacity for 'systems thinking' or 'systems leadership' is a developing concern in many public service organisations and governments, helping to formalise a concern about the fit between current organisational actions and the broader context in which these are situated. Hobbs (2019) provides a helpful overview of appropriate tools and approaches to help leaders engage their role from a systems perspective, spanning forms of systems mapping to participatory and dynamic approaches to planning, evaluation, and appraisal.

However, enhancing this capability requires more than changing how senior leaders think. Indeed, the epistemic and control barriers presented by outcome-focussed work make it impossible to coordinate effectively through the authority of existing system leaders. Leadership in a systemic perspective exists not in positions of authority, but in the relationships between actors, better conceived as Uhl-Bien et al (2007, p 306) argue as 'an emergent interactive dynamic that … emerges in a non-linear manner from interactive exchanges, or more specifically from the spaces between agents'. In this sense leaders play an important role in fostering coordinative capability by setting the conditions for leadership to emerge in other areas. Leaders also have an important directive role in setting a broad, inclusive, and motivating vision. Instead of 'closed loop' performance targets, principles, standards or a shared 'vision' may provide an appropriate model of organisational control, setting expectations while permitting sufficient fluidity in how local interpretations are created (French and Mollinger-Sahba 2021).

Because many coordinative challenges are both structural and systemic, it is likely that integrative structures need to be created to enable strategic cooperation across teams, departments, organisations, and sectors. Coordination between horizontally arranged entities (such as teams, departments or organisations) traditionally takes place on a continuum, from information sharing arrangements, to looser forms of cooperation, networks, or alliances, to more integrated models where processes, staff, and even budgets are shared (see McLoughlin and Wilson 2013). Such models of multi-agency working are by now well established in most OECD countries.

Notable approaches include structures like the multi-agency safeguarding hubs established in most UK local authority areas which have sought to improve information sharing and risk management by providing a 'one stop shop' for individuals to access support from a range of support agencies. Multi-agency coordination has also been promoted through service-level agreements and other forms of multi-party contracting and by integrating data into electronic shared records (McLoughlin and Wilson 2013). Basing contractual terms and payment on the demonstration of results is a prevailing orthodoxy, particularly in commissioned services. However, evidence suggests this can prohibit flexibility and collaboration by amplifying the management focus on data production rather than improvement (McLoughin and Wilson 2013, Wilson et al 2013, Cornford 2019, Jamieson et al 2020; French et al 2022). An alternative are innovations in relational contracting where contracting situations which are 'incomplete', that is, where the information, actions and interactions needed which cannot be attained or specified at outset and must evolve in response to identified needs. In this approach, contracting parties agree to become bound by a set of shared principles and priorities to govern behaviour and interaction, creating a form of shared and contextualised accountability and trusted relationships within a long-term collective endeavour.

There may be other cases where the frequency of interaction or degree of interdependency demands teams, departments, or organisations to become integrated rather than interconnected. One hopeful area is pooling budgets to share risk and systematise buy-in from participating parties.

Plymouth City Council's integrated commissioning model in adult social care has pooled four individual budgets into one single flexible budget, managed on a relational basis through an alliance contract (Lowe et al 2021b). Another example is the 'Bespoke by Default' approach being pioneered at Gateshead Council where the needs of the citizen are the starting point for a relationally-centred service approach drawing in a range of multi-agency service responses as necessary (see Smith 2020).

As the UN Sustainable Development Goals show, outcomes can still play an important coordinative role in performance regimes which are future-facing and feature distributed power relationships. Outcomes might function as cross-sectoral boundary objects and integrative structures which enable effective coordination in the absence of central direction (see French and Mollinger-Sahba 2021). Coordination capacity can be enhanced by models of collaborative performance management which span boundaries and work to develop shared expectations and dialogue across vertical organisational structures. Outcome-based 'wellbeing frameworks' (Wallace 2019), the Paris Agreement climate targets, or the UN's Sustainable Development Goals seek to mobilise actors around systemic goals far beyond the organisational boundary. While these are often convened by central organisations, they often operate through persuasion, influence, and negotiation rather than coercion and competition (French and Wallace 2022). Finally, performance measurement frameworks can facilitate opportunities for cross-boundary learning and sharing, with measures and indicators structuring collective sense-making processes and providing a shared language to facilitate coordinated action (Cornford et al 2013; Cornford 2019; French 2021).

Adaptive capability

Our CTOC situates public service professionals amid constant dynamism as changes in outcome systems occur at individual, community, or population-levels. Services and interventions must renew and update their activities to sustain their relevance to a dynamic external environment. Adaptation in complex systems is incorporated through forms of sense-making, learning, and adapting through feedback, a key process underpinning both self-organisation and emergence. Our third and final dynamic capability is therefore *adaptive capability*: the ability of public service systems to adapt to or pre-empt changes in their operating contexts.

One core theme of complexity-informed management scholarship is to position learning rather than control as a key engine of improvement (Mintzberg and Waters 1985; Bourne et al 2018). Adaptation can be pre-emptive, involving exploratory 'searching' mechanisms, for example through horizon scanning, contingency planning, or forecasting. In situations of uncertainty, however, opportunities for beneficial adaptation may be more feasible through reaction rather than prediction.

Such an approach would challenge organisations to repurpose corporate and HR functions from instruments of organisational control and accountability to those which facilitate learning and purposive adaptation. Strategists and planners might incorporate what Mintzberg and Waters (1985) call 'emergent strategy', in which observed performance involves strategising on a dynamic and ongoing basis. By keeping strategy provisional and tentative, decision making can proceed on a sense-and-respond basis better suited to complex environments (Kurtz and Snowden 2003). Models of transformational and adaptive leadership can facilitate such a learning-orientation through fostering the intrinsic motivation of staff and supporting a culture of responsible risk taking and tolerance to failure. Organisations might also sanction learning and adaptation through for instance commissioning pilots, experiments, or smaller-scale tests of change.

Revising and refining organisational processes and functions is doubtless important; however, our depiction of a dynamic, individuated outcome creation process requires adaptation on a more dynamic and devolved basis. Outcomes are, to use Heifetz et al's (2009) terms, not technical challenges to be resolved by better processes, but adaptive problems which can only be tackled with the active support of people 'with' the problem. The appropriate response is 'micro adaptation' (Heifetz et al 2009), a process driven by the creative energies of motivated, informed, and connected public service professionals. In this view, adaptation would occur through a dynamic process of co-creation between practitioners and service users, in which service capabilities are combined with an individual's own capabilities and relationships – support networks, skills, community assets, and other resources – to give the greatest potential to improve outcomes.

It is also important that adaptation is cyclical and fuels opportunities for broader organisational learning (Lowe et al 2021b; Lowe et al 2022). Processes identified by service professionals to impede value creation can be signalled for change, while the discovery of unmet needs could prompt exploration of new ways of working. Adaptive capability could be further enhanced by creating structures for learning and sharing beyond its site of origin – for instance communities of practice (Lave and Wenger 1991) or parallel organisational structures (Hawk and Zand 2014) which can connect learning from micro adaptation to higher-order organisational processes to institutionalise changes. The purpose of core functions like performance management might also shift from controlling workers to enact a pre-defined strategic plan, toward serving the informational needs of staff at multiple levels to make purposeful decisions and engage in informed navigation of outcome-focussed work. Critical approaches to performance management, such as Bourne et al's (2018) System of Systems approach or Jakobsen et al's (2018) Internal Learning model provide alternative schematic architectures for motivating improvement.

Summary

Building on Teece et al's (1997) dynamic capabilities theory we have described three core capabilities we consider essential in enabling public service systems to engage meaningfully with the complexity of outcomes:

- *Stewardship capability*: the capability of public service professionals to act as responsible stewards of publicly-valued outcomes.
- *Coordinative capability*: the ability to shape patterns of interaction to mobilise and integrate the knowledge, resources, and procedures necessary to improve outcomes.
- *Adaptive capability*: the ability of public service systems to adapt to or pre-empt changes in their operating contexts.

This set of capabilities offers an alternative design logic to the RTOC, and connects a public health view of an emergent outcome creation process across the policy-administrative divide. In our view, outcomes are improved not by a rationalistic optimisation of service efficiency, but by strategic investment in the dynamic capabilities of public service systems.

It is also important to recognise the limitations of this approach. We do not contend these three capabilities should be the sole concern of governments or public agencies. Our approach does not accommodate democratic values which are central to public value (Moore 1995) and which the government must uphold in addition to improving societal wellbeing. We recognise that many of the normative concerns which animate day-to-day working concerns within public agencies extend beyond a singular focus on the effectiveness of services. Public service professionals face overlapping policy directives, and multiple, potentially contradictory, accountability relationships with different stakeholder groups which must also be accommodated.

It is also important to note also that these capabilities relate most directly to the creation of social, health and psychological outcomes which are created and experienced by individuals. Environmental, cultural, economic, and democratic outcomes are also constitutive of social value and societal wellbeing (for example Heydecker et al 2022). Environmental outcomes relating to global heating also impact on people's wellbeing but are not lived by individuals or co-produced in the same way that social, health and psychological outcomes are. There are therefore multiple valid tradeoffs which policymakers and public service professionals must consider in addition to the concern which animates this book. Nevertheless, if public services fail to develop these requisite dynamic capabilities, we predict poor outcomes will be the result.

The three capabilities suggested here may serve an operational function as a self-assessment or appraisal tool for an organisation or initiative to assess its capability in meeting the demands of outcome-based working. For instance, an organisation could convene an organisation-wide conversation to assess its strengths and weaknesses against each capability or to assess readiness for change and focus for future investments. They might also provide an analytical frame for analysing the likely or actual consequences of public service reforms on social outcomes. A competitive tendering process which is found to initially cut costs, but to have done so through de-skilling and demotivating its workforce, could be judged to have worsened its capability for improving outcomes. Our primary purpose in this chapter, however, has been to ground our CTOC in a robust and accessible theoretical context, rather than to provide tailored guidance for practitioners. Connecting theory with practice is the subject which the following chapters will now address.

FIVE

Human Learning Systems: a new trajectory in public service reform?

With our distinctive appreciation of complexity and the identification of dynamic capabilities that support it, we now turn towards how these capabilities might be mobilised in the real world, and what the practical implications are for those seeking to address outcomes within a complexity frame. In this chapter we explore a novel approach to implementing a complexity-informed management practice in public and non-profit organisations, HLS (Lowe and Plimmer 2019; Lowe et al 2020a; 2020b; 2022; Lowe et al 2021b). We describe the principles of HLS and its genesis into a substantial service reform coalition involving more than 300 organisational members, drawing on evidence from a rich cohort of case studies. This chapter seeks to examine HLS as an applied model of public service reform which responds explicitly to the four complexities outlined in Chapter 3. The capabilities proposed in Chapter 4 are then applied in an analytical capacity to explore how HLS might meaningfully engage with this alternative worldview.

We highlight a strengths-based perspective implicit in HLS, which illustrates how reformers have harnessed agency, assets, and capabilities to purposefully embed more human, learning-oriented, and systemic practices in service contexts. The relational work involved in this is central to this examination and offers a lens through which we can understand the struggles, strategies, and investments involved in service reform practice in organisations and places. We inspect the HLS case study evidence closely to examine how far complexity frames of reference take us in understanding HLS practice.

Origins of HLS and basic theoretical components

Human Learning Systems is used to describe the emergent practice, ideas, and principles of many people and organisations who have been exploring complexity-informed approaches to commissioning, funding, leadership, strategic, organisational management, and service delivery alternatives to NPM. At the core of HLS is a concern for how organisations continually learn and strive to achieve value through emergence with a range of stakeholders through a 'Learning as a Management Strategy'. To understand value and outcomes while accounting for complexity means privileging human diversity, curiosity, and collaboration in how outcomes are created. Thus, the fundamental ethos of HLS espouse human agency, relationships, and flourishing as a moral purpose of public service, learning as a management strategy to ensure public services help people in their complex life contexts, and systems, not singular services of organisations, as the requisite unit of analysis for understanding how outcomes are created. To review HLS further, we take each element in turn.

The first is re-establishing the interests and needs of the 'human' in the design and delivery of services, to counter the corrosive effects of substituting life experiences with proxy indicators inherent in performance management and metric-focussed service design and performance management (Lowe and Wilson 2017; French et al 2021a). HLS views each person's life as a complex system and seeks not only to appreciate the experience of complexity through the lens of individuals and their relationships, but claims that this is necessary to establish any understanding of value in the context of each person's life as a complex system (Lowe et al 2022). The human element of HLS describes the individual focus for needs and outcomes, and how services can respond by drawing on their strengths, capabilities, and relationships with those they collaborate with, as well as those they co-produce service with. Finally, the human element articulates the nature of the networked 'human' work involved in complexity-informed service by recognising variety, building empathy, building an asset/strengths-based approach, and trusting that those serving in public and voluntary and community service organisations will act on intrinsic motivation (the public service ethos) to help and meet the needs of other human beings. To understand what counts as flourishing for each individual, and to be able to remain abreast of how that is continually re-articulated, means investment in a relationship and dialogue about these meanings, and also an appreciation that human need in its fullest sense falls significantly outside of the bounds of the current state provision of public service.

The second component, 'learning', has, in NPM approaches, been subverted by externally imposed performance management systems to support monitoring and reporting. These NPM agendas have demanded particular types of data which distort the storylines told to senior managers and regulators, thus equally distorting the potential for outcome data to tell real stories about real-life needs. HLS views learning as an emergent process of social innovation in response to local contexts (Lowe et al 2022). It also aligns with complexity theory's perspective that linear thinking in non-linear contexts will hinder learning by failing to account for feedback loops, effect delays (Sterman 2002), and the heterogeneity of human responsive behaviours. Those who have honed their descriptions of HLS practice also provided details of *how* they embed learning, inspired by approaches to action learning including appreciative inquiry, reflective practice, learning communities, and rapid learning cycles. In many cases iteration, experimentation, investment in learning capacity, and data usage for 'positive error cultures' are evident.

Finally, the 'system' element of HLS refers to how managers and practitioners perceive that outcomes are produced: to reflect the complexity of people's lives, public services cannot respond as single services and responses are inadequate if they are not continuously emergent. This dynamic, adaptive perspective on public services describes how heterogeneous agents and agencies within a particular context respond and adapt to the actions of each other, and in the case of public services, those they serve. Therefore, the work of HLS practitioners involves building relationships and trust between agents, and finding common ground, as well as acknowledging dissonance (Blackmore 2010), and exploring their 'system' together. One way of thinking about this is the idea of a 'system of interest' (Jackson 2019).

For HLS the 'system of interest' at any given time is the set of relationships which combine to afford or constrain the production of an outcome. Systems can be reflected (and linked) across various scales, all complex, from a person's life to an organisation, a place, or a country (Lowe et al 2021a). The challenge with this approach is the human and organisational limitations of being able to see the whole view. Therefore, in this chapter we will further explore what 'system' means in an HLS context and how this lens helps practitioners to govern complexity.

HLS has grown in scale and significance and become more expressive of the experiences of diverse case organisations who have 'experimented', reflected, and shared their stories. There is a certain 'real world' advantage and persuasion that HLS has over purely theoretical public management reform trajectories, which is established in its inclusive co-production process, embodied in the membership of the HLS Collaborative and in the co-writing of its recent report

(Lowe et al 2021b). What started out as a piece of research with 15 funders and commissioners, has since 2017 become a shared language used by policymakers and practitioners internationally to make sense of complexity-informed public management practice.

The case study approach to telling HLS stories

HLS has been informed by scholarly engagement with complexity in management and organisation theory, and by work in the application of complexity theory to public management (Pell et al 2016; Lowe and Wilson 2017; Pell et al 2020; French et al 2021a; Lowe et al 2021a). It is also a practice-informed approach which has been shaped by ongoing conversations which has so far involved over 300 commissioners, managers, and practitioners in a range of public service sectors, and with charitable funders, philanthropic organisations, and delivery organisations in the voluntary and community sectors. Co-production has increasingly been a core operating principle and expression of HLS in practice. Here we outline the approach taken to the production of the case study data, and to its analysis.

A narrative case study design was used to develop stories of practice from each case context. Case studies are purposefully designed as a method of capturing phenomenon in real-life contexts, and in the definition provided by Stake they can serve as 'both the process of learning about the case and the product of our learning' (Stake 1995). An organising group of HLS 'champions' (consultancy organisations, practitioner pioneers, and academics) was established to oversee the curation of these case studies. Invitations to write case studies were sent to 49 organisations known to the organising group for their pioneering work in September 2020. Case study authors were asked to use a template to ensure consistency in the key areas covered and members of the organising group were assigned to support case study authors based on pre-existing relationships and familiarity. Once the initial versions of case study drafts were written, consent was gained from each author to share with other members. A member of the organising group extracted data using an analysis template based on the HLS framework, and these were then shared with a second analyst which ensured consistency in the extraction of data. This process was also iterated, with certain elements modified for clarity, to put forth more information, or to sense-check interpretations.

Following this first round of analysis, we invited authors to share and read each other's case studies, to gain further insights and identify patterns to discuss at a sense-making session with all authors. The session was recorded, and a summary was circulated to support revisions. This iterative process of collective sense-making and co-writing built stronger shared narratives, identified the barriers and tensions encountered, and brought forward early indications of what had been achieved through adopting an HLS approach.

At the end of this process, 29 case studies were finalised and published in a public report (Lowe et al 2021b). This chapter has sampled these, along with an additional 10 accounts previously written by other organisations but using comparable templates. This case study material was self-submitted and written mainly from an organisational perspective, so was rooted in a process of reflective self-assessment. However, the methodology incorporated some degree of peer review with analysts in the organising group meeting monthly to discuss what patterns they were identifying from the written cases, sense-making sessions, and their own discussions, to produce an updated expression of HLS in the publication of an e-book: *Human Learning Systems: Public Service for the Real World* (Lowe et al 2021b).

Some of the case studies have been co-authored with 'learning partners' (Hesselgreaves et al 2021) from, among others, the Centre for Public Impact, Easier Inc., Collaborate, and Northumbria University. Therefore, the case studies we have drawn upon (see Appendix) include many whom the authors of this book have a long-term working relationship. All the interpretations presented here are subjective and heuristic.

Case studies

Each example of HLS in practice presents an emphasis in its narrative across the 'human', 'learning', and 'systems' elements. Figure 5.1 illustrates the heuristic structure used to analyse where case studies tend towards in their narrative emphasis. The examination presented here is a necessarily partial picture of an emergent practice, and not a definitive representation.

Where a case study's emphasis was balanced across more than one of these elements, that case study is plotted (with a star) somewhere between elements, depending on the extent to which each element features. Plotting the case studies this way enables us to discuss the merits of each element in the context

Figure 5.1: The template of HLS narrative case studies

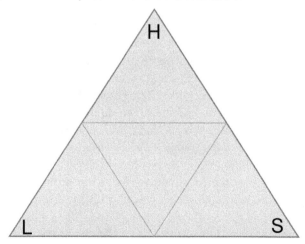

of complexity, capabilities, and perspectives on outcomes, as emphasisd by the narrative presented in the case studies.

Human stories as a lens for understanding value

First, we focus on those cases with descriptions of 'Human' assets and consider what this tells us about alternatives to outcomes-based performance management. The first observation is that this cluster of case studies shown in Figure 5.2 is characterised by third sector organisations: grass roots organisations, community interest companies, or in some other form community-led or community-situated organisations. The lack of statutory obligations may offer them affordances in their delivery which supports flexibility in responding to the variety of human need.

These cases adopt language that focuses on needs, stories, and struggle. The expression of need is usually with an emphasis on empowerment and equity 'emphasising those who have barriers to engagement' (Aberlour Child Care Trust)

Figure 5.2: Plot of 'human' narratives

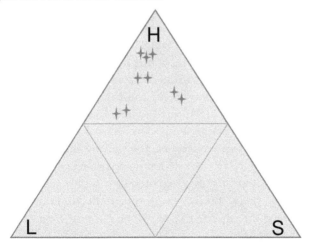

for all in the system including organisational staff. Moray Wellbeing Hub even considered equity as a key decider in choosing a Community Interest Company over a charitable organisational formation, as it reflected diversity and equity in their values. However, many of these organisations see needs that are fundamental and basic and respond with fundamental and basic provision: 'fridge and freezer, washing machines, clothing bank, library and family rooms' (Aberlour Child Care Trust).

Case studies which intentionally seek to break such strong and cyclic associations between situational factors accept the challenge that social problems are created by multiple, interdependent factors, and are usually socially entrenched, in line with compositional complexity. For others, this aligned more with experiential complexity, 'we "see" the individual and not just their needs' (Help On Your Doorstep). Because these perspectives on a flourishing life are so individualised, outcomes were similarly in flux, their creation characterised by 'no formal process ...' (IVAR evaluation report of Help On Your Doorstep). Storytelling was a common writing approach taken to compiling case studies when experiential content was at the forefront. Cases often described detailed accounts of decision making, informed by values, emergent behaviours, and often by intuition: 'Our story of change has developed in a much less schematic way, driven by intuition, a sense that we were doing the right thing (without always being able to articulate why, except that it was better and more honest than what others were doing) ...' (Coast and Vale Community Action).

What is particularly striking is the intertwining of the stories of the authors, their colleagues, and those of the communities they serve. In many cases, the authors chose to suspend their identity as professionals altogether: 'I can only help another person by being human and empathetic to him, I don't have to be an expert, like a psychologist to help another' (Vinarice Prison).

This focus on individuals, their experience of life, and the connection made between individuals and those in service conforms to experiential complexity, which acknowledges the unique experiences of the individuals encountering causal conditions and understanding what needs, strengths and priorities might inform a service response: 'Being human, working through trusting relationships and being committee to an ongoing process of learning and reflection often feels far from intuitive' (Aberlour Child Care Trust).

The narratives of need and struggle from all in the stories demonstrate a deeply held 'human' emphasis which may reflect the traditional missions of, and community-facing nature of voluntary and community sector organisations and highlight how this compassion-driven focus on experiential complexity can be at personal and emotional cost.

Table 5.1 shows how, as well as illustrating how different complexities are addressed by the human element of HLS and how needs are meet through establishing what is important to people, these cases also provide insight into what capabilities are being exercised. Drawing on the discussion in Chapter 4, stewardship capability seems most closely related, holding strong parallels with being trusted to operate based on values, ethics, and professionalism, rather than control.

Learning as strategic intent

Figure 5.3 positions a collection of case studies in which learning was a particular emphasis in their narrative. Learning as an established mode of organisational change is inherent in these organisational strategies, but it is notable how learning and working towards a positive error culture now makes its way into the mission statements and operational fabric of some:

Our purpose is to use the principles of Human Learning Systems to radically change the way we do things, to be a living example of what can be done when

Table 5.1: Human narratives as expressions of complexity and capability

HLS	Theme	Complexities for outcomes-based management (nature of the work)	Capabilities (nature of the capability)	Implications for outcomes
Human	Seeing and describing struggle and need, and public servants place themselves in this narrative	Experiential (variety and compassion work)	Stewardship capability (operate based on values, ethics, and professionalism, not control)	An individual's experience is the lens for understanding value
	Human needs are structurally linked	Compositional (public health work)		

we accept that being human is messy, we are making mistakes and learning from them continually and that our organisational system has to reflect that, rather than seeking to control what it can't really control anyway. (Empowerment)

As well as the expected contribution that learning has for enabling change, these cases offered detailed descriptions of learning which support two other strategic purposes. The first was using learning as a strategy to support and deepen relationships, and in turn, systemic wellbeing. This type of strategy prioritises more personalised experiences of learning as a social endeavour with wellbeing as a core concern. For example, Empowerment described how deeply personal and emotional learning work was, through their use of social pedagogy (Hatton 2013: Hämäläinen 2015). The Collective Impact Agency described how learning events were established specifically with a purpose for designing change, but became spaces which fostered relationship building: 'Slowly, the

Figure 5.3: Plot of human and learning narratives

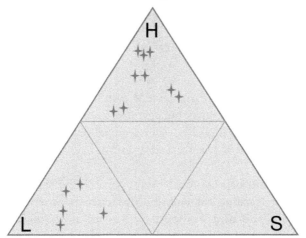

group came to the explicit realisation that prioritising the time to deepen the relationships was more important at this time than delivering a project that would be externally visible ... the collective decision to prioritise and dedicate time for relationship-building felt profound' (Collective Impact Agency).

Second, some used learning as a strategy for supporting the governance of systems change. Learning was often enacted as a formalised and in some cases proceduralised process. Although systems of learning used to support a governance strategy can produce impactful effects across the learning organisation and system, close attention should be paid to the potential risks of a learning system moving from a function of embedding learning for governance, to entrenching learning for an unexpected form of performance management. One community-based case study reported struggling with the creation of an organisational coaching system:

> within a governance or 'assurance' framework, robust enough to satisfy the rigorous regulatory environment in which it operated ... We felt as if we were drowning in the endless requests for evidence that our procedures were sufficient and the production of raw data to demonstrate compliance with targets and standards. (Neighbourhood Midwives)

This group was still required to serve an existing outcomes-based performance management system, highlighting the challenges for community organisations to enter into alternative accountability relationships. One national-level case study did implement a cross-place learning system:

> The value of a national body convening a space for shared learning on emerging practice is now being formalised and embedded into all ihub quality improvement and service redesign programmes ... as a

national improvement organisation, we recognise that the theoretical discourse on change and improvement can be intensely polarising with ongoing debates as to whether change is primarily driven through a focus on relationship and conversation or through a focus on process and system design. Our belief is that we need both as in real life the outcome is defined by a complex interplay between system/process design and people/relational issues. Accordingly, our improvement approach focuses on both the objective reality of process design and the more subjective world of relationships. (Health Improvement Scotland)

In addition to employing learning strategies in response to dynamic complexity and for relationship building, case studies also utilised learning strategies to navigate governance complexity by assembling multiple agents to coordinate around bespoke solutions to unique problems even in rigid external governance frameworks (though this endeavour appears easier for government learning systems with statutory obligations). Meanwhile, some cases remained assertive in paying close attention to the individualised experience of distinct outcomes, often focussing on sharing learning in real time about current problems and cases. Learning, then, operates across a number of complexities in layered configurations, supporting adaptive capability by catalysing change from action and reflection and by brokering learning relationships across external teams and organisations. These relationships are summarised in Table 5.2.

Investment in systemic relationships and learning to produce outcomes

Systems work is, so far, the most widely interpreted and least well-defined of the HLS elements described in the case studies. Cases which emphasised this element of HLS are shown in Figure 5.4. In HLS organisations, systems work refers to

Table 5.2: Learning narratives as expressions of complexity and capability

HLS	Theme	Complexities (nature of the work)	Capabilities (nature of the capability)	Implications for outcomes
Learning	Learning as a strategy for enabling change	Dynamic (learning infrastructure to create conditions for change)	Adaptive capability (adapting routines of work based on new information)	Learning is the mechanism by which unique human needs and relationships are embedded in strategic purpose, ensuring continual revision of outcomes
	Learning as a strategy to deepen relationships	Experiential (relational work)	Stewardship capability (understanding relationships as value-creating)	
	Learning as a strategy to support governance, processing and formalising sense-making about evidence and action	Governance (investment in trans-boundary learning)	Coordinative capability (constructing inter-organisational relationships as resources)	

Figure 5.4: Plot of human, learning and system narratives

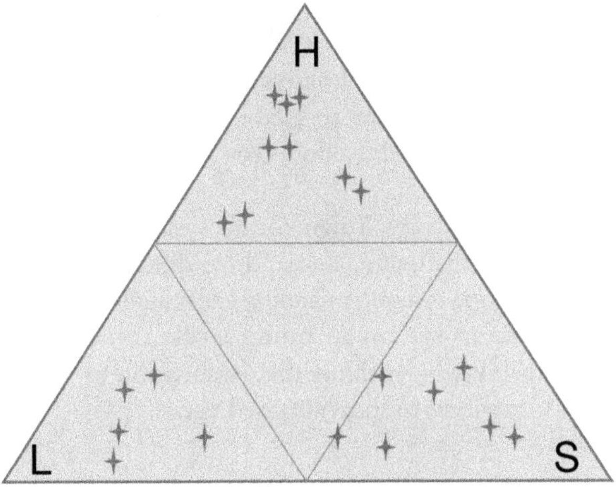

the unit of analysis to which purpose is applied (Lowe et al 2021b), and from which outcomes are produced. In the analysis presented here we can build on this by considering what resources systems provide, and what resources they need, to function as intended.

Most case studies were working within an austerity context where agency and resource constraints made systemic approaches challenging to establish. Some cases focussed on stitching parts of the system together by brokering relationships, although this did not always extend to involve external parties. As shown in strategy links closely with coordinative capability, but could also respond to both compositional and governance complexities by enabling different agencies to integrate resources to tackle shared social challenges:

> Originally the programme set out to achieve its aims of reducing social isolation and obesity by dividing its programme into 3 streams; the built environment, new models of care and community activation. Over time it became apparent to Bicester Healthy New Town

(BHNT) stakeholders that a systems-based approach was needed, as the value seemed to be added when the 3 streams interacted with each other ... BHNT developed its role as what the stakeholders are defining as a system connector ... In order to enable such interaction to take place. (Bicester Healthy New Town)

Bicester Healthy New Town found system convening to be its greatest challenge, demanding significant effort in 'understanding the system', including engaging in peer learning and undertaking system mapping work. This developed adaptive capability by enabling the organisation to recombine elements to respond to individualised needs.

Working in this way recognises that outcomes are produced by whole systems rather than individuals, organisations or programmes. Consequently, to improve outcomes, we need to work to create 'healthy' systems in which people can co-ordinate and collaborate more effectively utilising a strengths-based approach. This approach results in better experiences, better outcomes and it has potential to increase collaboration, enable innovation, build employee motivation, and deliver cost savings. (Liverpool City Region Combined Authority)

In several cases, such as Liverpool City Region Combined Authority, the Plymouth Alliance and Sobell House, the commissioner-provider relationship and contracting arrangements were redesigned based on a shared systemic understanding of purpose. These structural arrangements helped embed coordinational capacity at a system level and broker a broader range of resources to bear in tackling compositional complexity. These cases typically invested first in building collaborative infrastructure, however all also demonstrated a clear emphasis on inter-organisational learning within collaborative relationships. Table 5.3 summarises the

Table 5.3: System narratives as expressions of complexity and capability

HLS	Theme	Complexities (nature of the work)	Capabilities (nature of the capability)	Implications for outcomes
Systems	Coordination efforts of multi-agency inclusion as expressions of system behaviours	Compositional (collaborative work)	Coordinative capability (leveraging system resources)	Outcomes are created through the adaptive investment, provision, and use of collective resources, including learning resources
	Collaborative learning about systems	Experiential (relational work)		
	Funding and contracting learning at the systems level	Compositional (investment work)		

relationships between capabilities, complexities, and the system element of HLS.

The 'central cluster'

The cases used as exemplars of 'Human', 'Learning', and 'Systems' were chosen because of an emphasis in self-reported case studies of a particular element. Most case studies emphasised only one or two of the elements rather than all three. The HLS report (Lowe et al 2021b, p 100) claims that 'Human', 'Learning', and 'Systems' are so internally consistent that they are examples of each other: where we see one, we will find the others. However, we find this is not always the case: each case study faced unique challenges and articulated clear strengths with certain elements, but most often not all of them together. This may be a self-reporting bias, a lack of awareness, or perhaps it could represent an effect of prioritisation.

Here we examine the properties of a significant minority of case studies where descriptions of H, L, and S were more balanced (those denoted in the central quadrant of Figure 5.5. Here we examine what commonality those in the 'central cluster' – the oval in the central quadrant.

In addition to developing the capacities and capabilities discussed so far, cases in the 'central cluster' benefited from the compounding effects of investing in learning as a management strategy (Burnes et al 2003), which invariably included the appointment of, and in most cases co-authorship with a learning partner (Hesselgreaves et al 2021) (some called these actors 'thinking partners'). This involved brokering an externally facilitated learning process to 'hold uncertainty and complexity and communicate theoretical content' (Stirling Council and the Robertson Trust), enhancing adaptive capability by providing opportunities to reflect on learning and consider how it might inform change. Table 5.4 relates the characteristics of these 'central cluster' cases to the capabilities and complexities.

Figure 5.5: Complete plot of Human Learning System case narratives

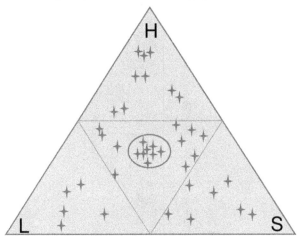

The investment in learning as a management strategy was apparent in other investment decisions, which devolved budgets to learning teams (for example Wellbeing Teams), financial investment in learning processes (for example Stirling Council and the Robertson Trust). This was also evident in these operational decisions and the conduct of decision making in senior leadership teams, which in several central cluster cases was based on what people had noticed about key metrics, collective analysis, and sharing successes and failures through their learning processes.

> The learning process is governed by everyone within Mayday who lives the learning culture of constant reflection and 'challenge and be challenged'. The process of listening, reflecting, challenging and changing is continuous and underpins all of our work. (Mayday Trust)

> Wellbeing Teams have demonstrated an ability to learn and adapt rapidly. Our self-managed model, emphasis on bringing the whole person to work, focus on self-care

Table 5.4: The 'central cluster' narratives as expressions of complexity and capability

HLS	Theme	Complexities (nature of the work)	Capabilities (nature of the capability)	Implications for outcomes
The Central Cluster	Investment in learning resource	Governance (investment in capabilities to make complexity governable)	Dynamic capability (stewardship, coordinative and adaptive capabilities together illustrate a dynamic value proposition where complexity is invested in, rather than minimised)	The practice of HLS is itse f in a wider infrastructure of resources which support the conditions for systems to produce outcomes
	Learning drives operations and decisions			

and use of technology to support and spread learning has made it possible for this to happen and for significant changes to roles and structure to be introduced quickly and effectively. Our handbook was rewritten six times in its first eighteen months to reflect the learning over that period. (Wellbeing Teams)

These cases offer an important insight into a strategic purpose not only focussed on improving practice, but on fostering the necessary conditions for coordinative, adaptive, and stewardship capabilities by investing in and embedding strategic learning processes. For some, this was experienced by steeping themselves in learning about systems thinking and complex systems approaches (The Children's Society). For others it was internalising a 'systems steward' role as their strategic approach to enabling systemic health (Wallsend Children's Community).

The 'central cluster' of HLS cases demonstrate that outcomes are produced as a result of deep systemic learning, which must be understood as a crucial strategic investment. Investment in learning capacity seems critical to develop the infrastructure and dynamic capabilities necessary to tackle systemic social change, and conversely, in enabling these dynamic capabilities and learning infrastructures to contribute to enabling an HLS practice to thrive.

Summary

In this chapter we sought to analyse how an emergent public sector reform community has responded to HLS and exhibited the dynamic capabilities required to initiate a trajectory *away* from an RTOC-orientation in management strategy. The relationships between the elements of HLS and the four complexities and three requisite dynamic capabilities we have developed in previous chapters are summarised descriptively in Table 5.5, and visually in Figure 5.6. HLS illustrates the potential for a public management practice where desired

Figure 5.6: HLS case narratives and their institutional environments

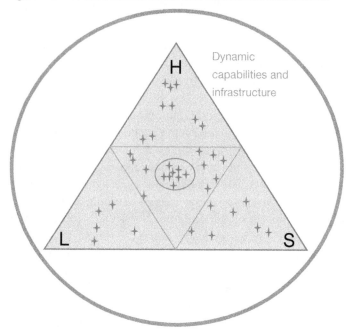

outcomes are viewed through a relational 'human' lens, delivered with learning as the mechanism through which needs and relationships are embedded in strategic purpose and capabilities, and supported by investment in a learning infrastructure, ensuring practice is responsive to the local challenges at hand. We have found that learning is often about relating (learning about people, learning with people about systems and from systems, learning from people about their stories), but that 'being human' (rather than delivering more technically efficient services) provided the motivation and momentum for a change in direction.

However, this exploration has highlighted that a wholesale HLS approach is more achievable in circumstances where funds and scope for influence/system leverage are present.

Table 5.5: Human Learning System narratives as expressions of complexity and capability

HLS	Theme	Complexities for (nature of the work)	Capabilities (nature of the capability)	Implications for outcomes
Human	Human needs are structurally linked	Compositional (public health work)	Stewardship capability (operate based on values, ethics, and professionalism, not control)	An individual's experience is the lens for understanding value
	Seeing and describing struggle and need, and public servants place themselves in this narrative	Experiential (variety and compassion work)		
Learning	Learning as a strategy for enabling change	Dynamic (learning infrastructure to create conditions for change)	Adaptive capability (adapting routines of work based on new information)	Learning is the mechanism by which unique human needs and relationships are embedded in strategic purpose, ensuring continual revision of outcomes
	Learning as a strategy to deepen relationships	Experiential (relational work)	Stewardship capability (understanding relationships as value-creating)	
	Learning as a strategy to support governance, processing and formalising sense-making about evidence and action	Governance (investment in trans-boundary learning)	Coordinative capability (constructing inter-organisational relationships as resources)	

(continued)

Table 5.5: Human Learning System narratives as expressions of complexity and capability (continued)

HLS	Theme	Complexities for (nature of the work)	Capabilities (nature of the capability)	Implications for outcomes
Systems	Coordination efforts of multi-agency inclusion as expressions of system behaviours	Compositional (collaborative work)	Coordinative capability (leveraging system resources)	Outcomes are produced through the adaptive investment, provision, and use of collective resources, including learning resources
	Collaborative learning about systems	Experiential (relational work)		
	Funding and contracting learning at the systems level	Compositional (investment work)		
The Central Cluster	Investment in learning resource	Governance (investment in capabilities to make complexity governable)	Dynamic capability (stewardship, coordinative and adaptive capabilities together illustrate a complexity value proposition where complexity is invested in, rather than minimised)	The practice of HLS is itself in a wider infrastructure of resources which support the conditions for systems to produce outcomes
	Learning drives operations and decisions			

The necessarily varied response to human strengths and needs means that HLS practice must be contextualised to a scaled-down system of interest, usually at a place-level. Some examples of HLS (the 'central cluster') signal that, although HLS seeks to help create conditions for better relational outcomes, the model by itself has certain conditional needs to flourish and become sustainable as a practice. These include investment in infrastructure and capabilities (asset-based dynamic capabilities, not just the funding and commissioning of practices or services) and the support for learning environments which allow for bespoke collaborative decision making and the institutionalisation of learning. This is partly to avoid reinventing the wheel – rationalist systems can reproduce themselves and crowd-out learning and emergent practice at the local level.

The data we have considered here (summarised in Table 5.5) is provisional and intended to generate discussion and debate rather than summative judgement about the success or not of HLS. Without an open process of reflection, debate, scrutiny, and dialogue about the struggle which its operating contexts present, HLS might well find its own philosophy of learning used against it, accused perhaps of not 'walking the talk'. Human, learning, system elements all help to mobilise a multi-faceted, polyphonic, and collective account of how public service can be delivered to promote improvement. This would be both across the spaces of citizen and staff wellbeing and flourishing inter-institutional relations in localities, and in some cases, a sustainable future for an alternative management practice seems to be in sight. However there remains much work for the researchers and practitioners involved to develop the potential of HLS further still, and provide critical assessments of how, and in which circumstances, an HLS approach can lead to better outcomes.

SIX

Learning partnerships: relevant research for a complex world

Our analysis of complexity poses a new organising question for scholars, managers, and practitioners alike: *how can public service systems be supported to build the requisite capabilities to manage the complexity demanded of them?* In this chapter, we approach this question from a research perspective, and discuss how a 'learning partnership' methodological approach between researchers and practitioners can support the development and elaboration of a complexity-informed practice. We draw on two substantive learning partnerships with UK charitable foundations – Lankelly Chase Foundation since 2017 and The Tudor Trust since 2018 – to discuss how this research approach can help public service organisations to build their dynamic capabilities.

Roots of a learning partner methodology

Organisational learning and professional learning are longstanding topics for educational and management research, informing notable approaches like Senge's (1990) 'learning organisation' as well as a large array of methods and tools, including appreciative inquiry (Johnson and Leavitt 2001), action learning sets (Boydell and Blantern 2007), and learning communities (Wilson et al 2023).

However, as public sector practitioners and managers seek to develop their practices, in a shift away from NPM to complexity-informed practice or a wider systems approach, they require additional capacity to scaffold the ability to learn through processes of experimentation (Easterby-Smith 1990). This in turn creates a space for consultancy and/or academic research work to develop this practice and the evidence for exploring what works, how and why in a given situation. One of the ways of framing this is through a process of action learning action research (ALAR). The ALAR approach advocates for a role of 'critical friend' as a way of creating a learning relationship between parties with the aim of fostering the role of an academic in a change–action process and the role of consultant as the change agent (Reason and Torbert 2001; Zuber-Skerritt 2002).

In our own academic engagement with organisations seeking to improve their fit with complex settings, we have at times been called on to perform as a 'learning partner' – a role whose objective is to facilitate learning processes, rather more traditional models of academic-practitioner knowledge creation like contract research, evaluation, knowledge exchange or research dissemination. This role conforms to the formalisation of HLS which, in common with many other complexity-engaged discourses, models and tools, identifies learning as a core engine of system change.

Buffardi and colleagues have found that the aim of integrating learning into programmes and organisations is considered common practice, yet a formal role of 'learning partner' (LP) is not yet widespread (Buffardi et al 2019; Hesselgreaves et al 2021), and research literature on 'learning partnerships' occupies a relatively small part of the much wider field of action-oriented research methods (French and Hawkins 2020). The concept of an LP is closely linked with existing approaches like the embedded researcher (Mickan and Coates 2022) or researcher in residence (Vindrola-Padros et al 2019), in bringing closer connection between academics and practitioners than is present in traditional social research, although LPs can be a more flexible approach than these methodologies (Hesselgreaves et al 2021). LP also links to 'engaged scholarship' (Van de Ven 2007) as the intention is to collaborate on complex issues in context, and the role is not of a consultant/academic expert who 'knows the answer' but as a researcher who aims to collaboratively co-produce further understanding.

Learning partner (LP) is not a new term, and many organisations use this to describe a complexity-informed approach to knowledge creation and mobilisation. There are examples of LP being used by independent institutes and consultancies, such as the Institute for Voluntary Action Research, Research for Real, the Centre for Public Impact, and Collaborate CIC, among many others, although practices range widely and there are few agreed principles for fulfilling such a role (see Hesselgreaves et al 2021). These partnerships tend to focus on practitioner-based learning in context, using techniques such as 'mirroring' and 'windowing', rather than the wider endeavour of knowledge and theory testing. From our perspective we distinguish between two orientations or styles of learning partnering, neither one better than the other, but with different characteristics. The first of these are Consultancy-orientated LPs which can provide opportunities for organisations to engage with rapid cycles of learning, which are primarily focussed on client needs and individual contexts through rapid reflection. On the other side are Academic-orientated LPs who might support longer learning cycles through recourse to knowledge creation in relevant fields by drawing patterns and themes into a broader academic discourse at an institutional or partnership frame in a form of slow-reflection. Both types of LP can work together with organisations to support and embed learning so that it becomes part of policy and practice.

Learning partnerships utilise a range of methodologies and methods. Approaches such as collaborative action research (Bennett and Brunner 2022), participatory action research (Kemmis et al 2014), action learning (Revans 1982), and action science (Argyris et al 1985) provide methodological processes for involving researchers in practice-shaping inquiry. Co-production (Durose and Richardson 2015), co-creation, and co-operative inquiry conversely engage practitioners in the design of core elements of the research process, ensuring that practice-relevant needs are taken on board and extending ownership of the research process. Although there are distinctions within each tradition, often in terms of methods and processes used, the approaches are 'loosely-linked' (Weick 1976) as a broad field of 'action-oriented' research roles, methods and tools which seem conceptually appropriate to the responsive, iterative, and engaged research demands of a complexity-informed public service praxis (French and Hawkins 2020).

Our approach to learning partnerships

We define a learning partnership as a connection between academic researchers, practitioners, and anyone else who is involved in innovating public services (such as independent researchers and consultants), where the intention is to learn with and from each other (Hesselgreaves et al 2021). Since 2017, we have played two key learning partner roles: for Lankelly Chase Foundation's Place Action Inquiry, and for The Tudor Trust's 'Funding and Commissioning in Complexity' action research project, as well as engaging in three further learning partnerships in a less extensive role.

Lankelly Chase Foundation (LCF) engaged us as a learning partner on their emerging place-based approach to system change to support them in a process of action inquiry. In this original role we worked both with the LCF staff team to explore the role of a funder and also with their partners in place to reflect on their work and to build collective understanding of LCF's emerging process (Lowe and French 2018). A broad-based learning framework was co-developed with LCF staff to describe the learning roles involved in this inquiry, building on Reason and Torbert's (2001) action research/action learning framework, which involved first person (self-reflection), second person (mutual inquiry in groups), and third person inquiry (engaging in wider research and practice on place-based systems change).

The Tudor Trust funded a three-year action research project on innovating funding and commissioning practice away from a rationalist approach to one which was complexity-informed. Tudor were subsequently enlisted, along with a number of other case studies, to embark on a learning journey to reflect on and make changes to their own learning practice. Drawing on the method used by the learning partnership already underway with Lankelly, our research role became an opportunity to support learning as part of a multi-stakeholder group (staff and trustees at Tudor, organisations which Tudor funds, and external consultants).

Supporting dynamic capabilities through learning partnership

Throughout this book we have referred to three dynamic capabilities required for working in complex environments. We use these capabilities as a broad framing to elaborate on our experiences on the benefits of a learning partnership approach, the barriers which might be encountered, and the methodological decisions we have made in order to improve our practice.

Stewardship capability

Stewardship capability, in the context of this chapter, relates to keeping the 'mission' of the work alive in the day-to-day work of practitioners, working to create and reinforce a common purpose, strengthening trust and relationships, and promoting and prioritising learning as a valued practice. LPs also have a role in curating learning flows – in the context of HLS, LPs support System Stewards to govern interconnected learning cycles connecting multiple system scales (Lowe et al 2021b). LPs can increase opportunities for learning by both championing the role of learning as an organisational priority, and providing structured support to the learning process. This may also have the benefit of the creation of an embedded learning practice which remains in the system when an LP relationship ends.

As learning partners for Tudor, we were able to prioritise learning through the creation of a 'learning group' which met every month for a year and focussed attention on developing funding practice through taking an HLS approach. The meetings intended to create a 'safe space' to reflect genuinely on the challenges of practice, rather than become a performative exercise. In both LCF and Tudor Trust cases, we helped share learning across levels of the organisation in a process of action inquiry (Reason and Torbert 2001). In The Tudor Trust, examples involved staff being encouraged to write a learning diary, and to engage in one-to-one discussions with a member of the research team (first person learning), the provision of two 'learning events' which included participants from the organisations that Tudor fund (second person learning), a peer learning group for grant managers (second person learning), and participation in a large-scale online webinar series on funding and commissioning practice (third person learning). The action inquiry was built into management practice with LPs stewarding the governance of distributed learning and staff given dedicated time and support to take part.

One risk which emerged in both cases is that responsibility for learning is 'outsourced' to the learning partner, with practitioner organisations in effect absolving themselves of the responsibility for learning. Some practitioners expected the

LP to neatly capture and package up learning, into a palatable format with little need for active engagement or reflection. In some cases this mirrored a traditional consulting or Continuous Professional Development (CPD) role, whereby academics became considered the 'experts', tasked with leading partners in the learning process. However, at times, this reduced the quality of interaction and organisational ownership of learning, with learning becoming little more than a transaction between researcher and practitioner.

From our other engagements it emerged that LPs, as a relatively novel approach to research practice, can also become mired in ambiguity. Practitioners at times became unable to comprehend what the role and remit of a LP is or should be, with engagement and commitment to learning becoming deprioritised. There were also at times evident mistrust which prevented honest reflection with LPs or colleagues. A few organisations became confused over what our role was, and either expected us to become firmly embedded within their organisation (which would have been an untenable resource constraint), or to play a limited functional role of 'expert or consultant' in efficiency-oriented actions. Taking this approach assumes a transactional approach to organisational learning with the LP essentially surrogating for organisational capability.

We have sought instead to develop a relational approach with our partners, where we spend time building relationships with participants, and understanding their unique, experiential perspective of working in complex social systems. Initial conversations about role expectations could involve both parties co-designing what the LP role would look like and managing expectations about shared commitments to it. We have also engaged in multi-level critical conversations with other learning partners (through part of an HLS collaborative learning group), and by employing our own learning partner who has supported us in strategic action and decision making on our LP journey. Clearly there is a 'sweet spot' or balance in the relationships between learning partners and the contexts in which they are working and this is likely to require ongoing work throughout a cycle of engagement which to an extent should remain equivocal. One of the practices that we believe supports this has been likened to a 'therapist's therapist' model of learning, where LP practitioners ought to be part of their own cycles of reflective learning (Buffardi et al 2019; Hesselgreaves et al 2021).

Coordinative capability

Coordinative capability relates to the need for mobilising and integrating the required resources, skills, and knowledge from independent actors to contribute to improving outcomes. This requires coordinated working across agencies to strengthen relationships, develop a common purpose, respond to problems, mobilise resources, and perhaps most crucially, enable opportunities for cross-organisational learning.

Learning partners are well positioned to support cross-organisational collaboration, and can often take the role of 'boundary spanners' (Needham et al 2017) across organisations by supporting iterative learning loops as part of an action research process (Argyris and Schön 1996). As learning partners we have coordinated cross-organisational learning through creating platforms and convening groups, using methods like learning circles, communities of practice, learning communities, and larger-scale learning events. This enables practitioners and academics to engage with different levels of learning including individual, peer and the wider research, thus enabling deeper reflection and reflexivity than when simply learning at the local level. These processes of learning have also fostered the development of relationships and trust, which we have found (in Chapter 5) to be important in improving collaborations working on systems change initiatives. At the same time, to reduce myopia, LPs may bring knowledge and perspectives which widen, or challenge, practitioners' knowledge base so that practice is not bounded simply by what is local (Reason and Torbert 2001).

Another core role we played in both LP roles was to help practitioners make sense of evidence, experiences and relevant concepts and theories to revise mental models, schema, and operating principles. LPs taking an action research/action learning process can therefore support further understanding of context, in order to make better-informed decisions (Phelps and Hase 2002; Piggot-Irvine et al 2015). This approach to learning stands in contrast to more object-oriented and reductionist forms of learning often engaged by academics and consultancies, where learning is often equated to a one-off training event, or form of continuous professional development, and thus can become an 'add-on' rather than an integral part of a formative approach to practice. Instead, LPs are potentially able to provide a bridge between research and practice, and thus this changes the nature of a more 'traditional' commissioned research or evaluation project to one which is more open-ended and adaptive to context and need.

However, there are associated barriers to taking a coordinative approach. Action research and cross-organisational collaboration are time and resource-consuming processes for both researchers and other participants (Badham and Sense 2006; Buffardi et al 2019). Resourcing an LP to do coordinative work can also be problematic, rewarding funders and larger organisations rather than smaller groups or less senior officials where support with learning may be more needed, particularly in times of fiscal restraint and budget cuts.

We have also found time to be a significant barrier to the research, with practitioners we have been working with citing this as a constraint to engaging fully in the research process. This has meant limited engagement in meetings and learning groups, often at the organisational level; cross-organisational events are usually better attended. Our reflection is that citizen-facing practitioners are less likely to attend and participate in the research due to the less predictable nature of their work and lack of priority given to learning opportunities compared to managers. Gatekeeping behaviour has also been a feature of LP projects, which can stall action research projects and prevent broader based participation (Bennett and Brunner 2022).

As well as having time and resources to be able to take part, practitioners also need to be motivated to participate in research, and personal motivations and bias will come into play with impact on levels of engagement (Buffardi et al 2019). Furthermore, the quality of action-oriented research may continue to be seen as being inferior to scientific-objectivist research, and approached with caution due to the open-ended nature of projects (Bennett and Brunner 2022). All factors have played a part in reducing engagement from practitioners in our experiences.

It has taken many years to build relationships with the case studies, and while we can claim some success, there are also many cases which have not flourished. The reasons for this have sometimes been out of our control, such as practitioner overload, through for example, multiple learning experiments being trialled simultaneously. There has also been reticence from others who do not see the value in engaging in academic work of any type, and due to resource constraints and geographical distance, we struggled at times to build or retain shared intent to pursue learning trajectories.

Adaptive capability

Adaptive capability relates to how organisations explore alternative ways of working, learn and adapt existing routines. One key way LPs can develop this is by supporting practitioners and organisations to follow a reflective process which stimulates reflection and informs future planning and decision-making processes. The LP role might then play a role in knowledge mobilisation and integration by helping forms of evidence (be this scientific or experiential) find their way into everyday usage.

In our LP roles this was often challenging, and we had more success grounding theoretical concepts productively with senior organisational leaders than with practitioners. For example, both the HLS framework and the Lankelly Chase Learning Framework often met with mixed responses from practitioners, despite being partially grounded in their own experiences. Some claimed that frameworks lacked prescriptive detail and were too abstract to be useful. Others took the opposite opinion, that those same frameworks were too rigid and inflexible, and constituted a 'top-down' approach to the learning and change process. This resulted in members of one learning group feeling like they were being monitored and observed like 'fish in a bowl' – that they had to stick rigidly to an approach they had little say or stake in.

Throughout our LPs work we strived to pursue research which would be relevant for practitioners, and this often required taking a more participatory approach to the process. We found it helpful to conceptualise learning as a social phenomenon which could only be curated rather than something which to be extracted from its site of practice and managed into changes at the organisational level. Our own LP practice shifted toward a problem-oriented approach, starting the learning process with the concrete problems encountered by the practitioners (rather than external theory, concepts or models adopted by senior leaders or prescribed in professional codes or government legislation), and taking an inductive and pluralist approach with a variety of learning methods to fit different preferences. To prevent the process from becoming overly introspective, we as LPs took on responsibility for convening multi-agency practitioners working across different organisations into social learning forums, which prompted more genuine practice-changing adaptation in both cases.

As LPs we were embedded across multiple sites of organisation and could generate a holistic perspective on the key problems, relationships, and opportunities. This also afforded us privileged access to the whole process of organisational learning from when problems were first explored or ideas were generated by individuals, to how these eventually took hold at an organisational level through the formalisation of new language or understandings, or in policy change or the enactment of key strategic decisions. In the LCF case, key roles like 'associate', 'coordination team', and even 'learning partner' we used originally in dialogue with the organisation to describe new developments which gave bounding and context to a programme of work which had been extremely fluid and dynamic.

Work in LCF required us to operate in a variety of roles such as action researchers, detached social scientists, critical friends, work coaches and even mentors. Reflecting on our own approach, our identities as 'researchers', 'colleagues', or even 'co-creators' were often in flux, determined by the quality of relationship held with individual practitioners, and by the particular needs of the organisation at a given point in time. Our work as LPs for LCF began as a loosely organised action inquiry with a highly exploratory focus; however as practitioners themselves took on responsibility for learning and adapting, our role evolved to concern convening groups of practitioners and analysis of higher-level themes. Our role eventually morphed into a more traditional type of social science research as key elements of organisational mission developed the solidity to benefit from this (French et al in press). Effectiveness in building adaptive capability seems then to demand a corresponding flexibility, reflexivity, and ambidexterity from LPs and the institutional contexts in which they work.

Conclusion

This chapter has drawn evidence from our two main LP roles to illustrate some of the main benefits and challenges in helping organisations to develop the dynamic capabilities we have previously described. We have outlined how LPs can leverage coordinative capability through the co-production of learning infrastructure across organisations and systems, support stewardship capability through the cultivation of a learning culture, and adaptive capacity by providing flexible and ambidextrous support throughout as needs change.

Playing an LP role as an academic organisation has not been easy or straightforward, and we have found both sides of these partnerships have at times struggled to work productively in what can feel uncomfortably ambiguous and uncertain territory. We also draw attention to certain landmines: becoming an outsourced 'learning support' provider in effect absolving the host organisation of learning responsibility, or devolving into a transactional learning process concerned with the packaging and administration of learning for managerial purposes.

Although we have primarily focussed on the practitioner perspective, LPs can also bring advantages from an academic perspective. We were given unfettered access to organisational life, and had the resources and freedom to actively engage with emerging issues to break new scholarly ground. Set amid a steadily growing interest from the university sector in impact, community engagement and academic citizenship, learning partnership ought to prove fertile ground for change-oriented academics and consultants and the practitioners, managers and organisations they work with.

More broadly 'learning partnering' is an emerging methodology to assist public sector practitioners, commissioners, and managers to drive complexity-informed service reform. It has an associated set of practices which help those exploring the approach make informed choices when deciding how to support themselves when taking the necessarily reflexive approach to reform. However, as we have discovered through our work these relationships are by their nature ambiguous with tensions arising from the new ways of working between the various stakeholders with no one right way forward (Badham and Sense 2006; Hesselgreaves et al 2021). Notwithstanding these qualifications, LPs offer a conceptual frame which speaks to the complexities faced by public and non-profit sector practitioners, managers, and their organisations when working through the paradoxes and contradictions of change. It highlights that complexity-informed public management requires relationships that offer sustainable learning capacity not merely for individual organisations, but also for improvement and change within wider systems, communities, and landscapes of public management practice. It will take further research and more critical analysis of completed learning partnerships to better understand these challenges.

SEVEN

Harnessing complexity for better social outcomes: a reform and research agenda

> There is scarcely a single duty of government which was once simple which is not now complex. Government once had but a few masters; it now has scores of masters. Majorities formerly only underwent government; they now conduct government. Where government once might have followed the whims of a court, it must now follow the views of a nation.
>
> Woodrow Wilson (1887, p 200), *The Study of Administration*

This book has explored a problem which has animated governments and academics for more than a century: in an increasingly complex world, how can public services and social interventions create and sustain positive social outcomes for the people and populations they serve? As Wilson's remark shows, we are not the first to ask this question and will be far from the last. Yet this seems a question which must be *re-asked* in each era where the simplifying tendencies of government begin to confound its capabilities.

Readers of this book will hopefully understand, and perhaps know from their own work, that any sustainable response requires us to face up to complexity, rather than invoke past managerial tendencies to simplify, externalise, or ignore it. We hope our book provokes critical thinking and provides useful guidance for those seeking positive change in public and non-profit services.

We argue that in the human and relational services, outcomes are improved and value is created by investing in the requisite capabilities to manage the innate complexity of public service work. Our CTOC structures this challenge across four dimensions of complexity:

- Compositional complexity, which results from the interdependence and inter-determinacy of causal systems from which outcomes emerge.
- Dynamic complexity, which results from the volatility and flux of interacting causal factors and their operating environment.
- Experiential complexity, which results from the variety of ways in which outcomes are experienced and navigated by individuals.
- Governance complexity, which results from the distribution of knowledge, agency and resources needed to tackle outcomes across a range of independent actors.

Using the CTOC as a design guide and building on the dynamic capabilities approach of Teece et al (1997), we describe three dynamic capabilities – stewardship capability, coordinational capability, and adaptive capability – which together provide a strategic focus for building complexity-capable public service systems.

This new theoretical perspective provides more solid footing for understanding, designing, and appraising outcomes-focussed services and interventions. It outlines a novel service reform trajectory with distinct conceptual advantages relative to the current rationalist orthodoxy, particularly in the human and relational services. It also marks out a productive space for motivated researchers to take on a developmental role through action-oriented approaches like learning partnering. Figure 7.1 sketches out a working model of the key relationships between these components.

The destination we arrive at is not at a polished framework or a directive operating procedure for practice, but a broad theoretical perspective which might be adapted, extended or challenged by the insight of others. We do however argue this leads to a radically different reform trajectory than the current mainstream. We have shown how an RTOC has governed how outcomes are conceptualised, targeted and pursued, and has only grown more prominent as public administration evolved from traditional public administration to the NPM and into the current era of governance. While promising better accountability, a stronger incentive system, and to reset social intervention on an objective basis, this model has struggled to get off the ground without making fundamental methodological concessions or generating counteractive performance paradoxes. From our theoretical perspective, this model misdirects energy and resources, focussing on transactional capacity rather than dynamic capability. Viewed in this way, RTOC-derived approaches may well *reduce* the dynamic capabilities needed to improve outcomes.

As the outcomes agenda in public service reform gathers pace, it approaches a fork in the road. Do we continue to use outcomes as a technocratic apparatus to simplify and commodify public service – or chart a different approach based on a meaningful engagement with its inherent complexity?

And where might this latter course of action lead? One approach is to consider the principle of dynamic capability as a design framework in the construction, management, and appraisal of services and interventions. Initiatives in the human and relational services like the lauded Buurtzorg model for community care appear successful at least in part because its self-managing teams and organisational structure support

Figure 7.1: Building complexity-capable public services: a working model

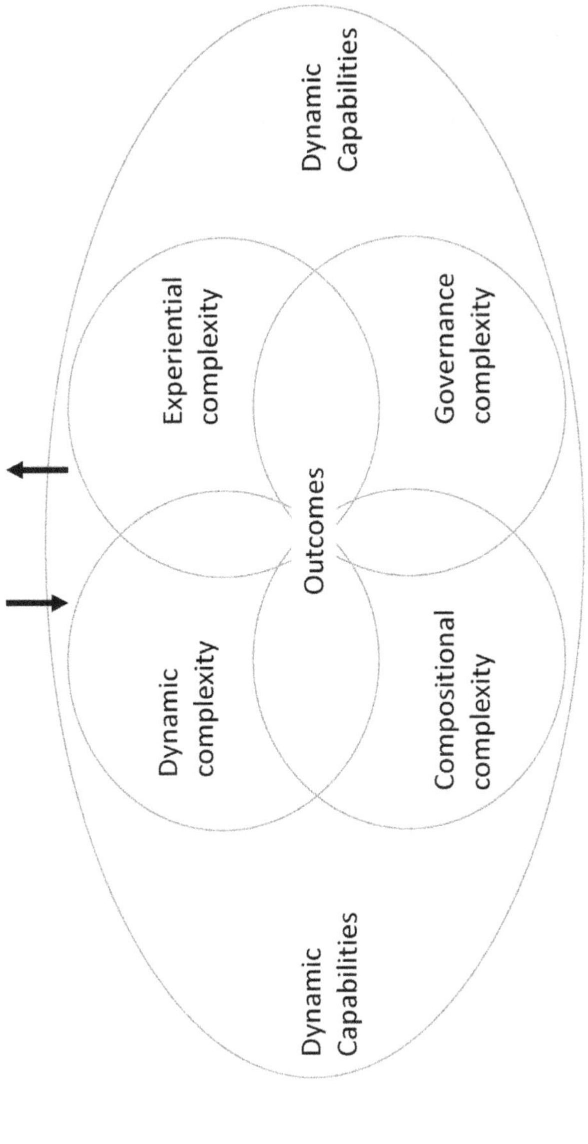

Learning Partnering

Dynamic Capabilities

Experiential complexity

Governance complexity

Outcomes

Dynamic complexity

Compositional complexity

Dynamic Capabilities

these capabilities. Conversely, our approach might be used as an evaluative frame to assess and perhaps even recondition the 'rationalist' models we have discussed, like outcomes-based contracting arrangements, for instance, based on their impact on dynamic capabilities.

While we have presented our theoretical perspective as an evolution in public service reform, others might understand it more as an attempt to revive what has been lost. In many respects the capabilities we describe were embedded in the trust and autonomy afforded to public service professionals under traditional public administration, which were subsequently eroded through NPM reforms (Freidson 2001; Radin 2006). For some scholars, the virtues of professional autonomy could be revived and updated in a modern governance context through a 'neo-Weberian' public administration (Pollitt and Bouckaert 2017) in which the dynamic capabilities we have outlined become accommodated through an extended and more flexible rule-based professionalism.

As we have previously noted (French and Lowe 2018), the transition from rationalism to complexity can instead be positioned as a Kuhnian paradigm shift, where the accumulating and irresolvable anomalies of the RTOC prompt a transition toward a different worldview and organising basis. For some, particularly those we have engaged in policy and practice in the UK, this theoretical perspective does feel like a fundamentally different reform trajectory. This is the position taken by HLS as an organising framework to socialise practitioners and policymakers in the unfolding of a reform agenda. However, whether what we present should be understood as a new paradigm, a more pragmatic design guide or a revivified and updated 'Neo-Weberian' state matters little to the real world.

So what about Amy, the council tax debt arrears case we reported in the introduction? As we described, the traditional approach to dealing with people in council tax arrears like Amy would be to send reminders, threats, and sanctions to coerce payment. Yet this is not what happened.

Alex had been granted more agency than equivalent managers in other local authorities. He prioritised time with Amy around his own caseload to listen to her and win her trust. He began to piece together reasons for past non-payment. Amy told Alex about her precarious work situation, her zero-hours contract and the instability which prevented her making past payments. He came to understand how her previous experience with the council and with bailiffs had driven her out of engagement and ruined her trust in public institutions – so Alex gave her his own work phone number to contact directly.

Alex understood that many of Amy's challenges would be beyond his own ability to resolve, however he knew how to pull in support from other council departments like social care, or even with the support of senior management from external agencies like the local housing association. He was able to hold back organisational procedures for reclaiming debt which he judged would just make things worse.

Through open conversation and negotiation, Alex and Amy were able to establish a payment plan which was successfully met in the three subsequent months. From the council's perspective, Amy's case met with a positive outcome. Alex, however, was more worried. He had not heard from Amy for some time, and became concerned that payments would soon drop off again.

The story we chose to start and finish this book is not one of resounding and unqualified success. Instead, it seems far more typical of the many we hear from people struggling to make public service capable of navigating complexity. The road to better outcomes seems longer, and the setbacks hit harder and feel more personal. Yet the thought of returning to what came before – a rational and efficient procedure of threats and sanctions in Amy and Alex's case – is unthinkable. Harnessing complexity gives public servants a fighting chance at improving lives.

On balance we would argue that, if carefully and critically managed, harnessing complexity should lead in aggregate to better social outcomes at reduced long-term cost to the public sector. However, our early experience also shows there remains substantial work in symphonising the theoretical implications of the CTOC with the practical reality of a resource-constrained, fragmented, and politically contested public service landscape.

Kuhn (1962, p 10) argued that successful new paradigms must be both 'sufficiently unprecedented to attract an enduring group of adherents away from competing modes of scientific activity' and 'sufficiently open-ended to leave all sorts of problems for the redefined group of practitioners to resolve'. Taking this advice, we end this book by posing five organising questions which might animate and sustain a critical collective inquiry in navigating this emerging possibility space in public service reform. These are *the accountability question*, *the assurance question*, *the unintended consequences question*, *the pragmatism question*, and *the research question*.

The accountability question

Our discussion clearly problematises a results-based accountability model based on individualised and linear attribution. However, accountability is a crucial and inextractible component of democratic governance and as close to a sacred virtue as exists in public administration. How can we make sure that engaging with complexity does not lead to a de-emphasis, or worse still, a deficit of accountability? On this point, there are many avenues which might be explored.

One is to transition from accountability to a position of legitimised trust in the motivations and expertise of public service professionals. Romzek and Dubnick (1987) describe a model of 'Professional accountability' which justifies an 'earned autonomy' through achievement of recognised standards and adherence to professional codes of practice. Accountability becomes regulated by internal mechanisms like professional associations and peer review, and an implicit social contract based on public consent. However, professional accountability is dependent on public trust and clear role expectations, both of which have gradually rolled back since NPM. There are also those like Radin (2006) notes who may use professionalism as a cloak to avoid accountability.

Another approach might be to change the direction of accountability from vertical (principal-agent) to horizontal models of peer or competency-based accountability. In this approach, members of a particular community become accountable to one another through collectively upheld and validated values and standards of competency. Critics might caution that horizontal modalities of accountability, however, may re-create their own counteractive norms and insularity, and lack responsiveness to external demands of social accountability.

Another proposed solution is to move the focus of accountability from results to learning. In this approach, actors would become answerable for the quality of learning (which is likely to include mistakes and missteps) rather than claims to impact. This holds the conceptual advantage of emphasising the primacy of learning as a driver of improvement, however it, too, faces conceptual problems. Learning is a personalised journey driven by intuition and determined by context. This may lead to particular difficulty in assigning blame or liability given learning is a virtue in its own right. For Bächtold (2021) the 'peculiar conflation of accountability as learning … legitimizes self-referential expert rule' and so marginalises accountability to citizens and service recipients.

One promising area for further research is how different modalities of accountability (for example horizontal, trust-based, learning-based or mutualistic and dialogic) can surrogate for traditional results-based accountability. However, each modality seems encumbered by its own set of problems. Practitioners should also be alert to creating new means of performativity in public service, and in preserving a critical democratic accountability beyond a self-referential commitment to do better.

Pragmatics intervene here, too. Accountability is not often a choice – nor does any single modality sit within a vacuum. Public managers are held to account by multiple stakeholders for often competing criteria, and must therefore prioritise certain commitments over others. How then can complexity-relevant models of accountability avoid being deprioritised by accountability demands from external principals?

In an era of declining trust there may be greater public value in privileging the normative dimension of accountability above its functional role in service effectiveness. While failure is inevitable in situations of uncertainty, it also seems necessary that a 'straight story' can be given to citizens who might seek redress or demand answers. How then might complexity arguments can be communicated to the public, and squared with cultural norms of democratic accountability? A realist view would be that demands for democratic accountability must be, at times, grudgingly reconciled with demands to cope with complexity. A pragmatic goal therefore might be to determine a model of accountability which is a workable compromise in both democratic and functional terms.

The assurance question

We have argued that the complexity of outcomes requires that public agencies invest in the dynamic capabilities of public service systems. 'Investment' here implies a commitment of time, effort and financial resources, and an assurance process to build confidence for decision making and account for risks involved. Decision-makers confront endemic uncertainty in our CTOC. How then can assurance be provided to help people initiate and deepen their service reform journeys?

This will strike some as beginning with the wrong question – leaders should have the vision and courage to set an ambitious agenda and sanction appropriate reforms even in the absence of a straightforward assurance process. Indeed, many HLS case studies have relied on senior leaders taking the initiative and providing an authorising environment for risk taking in their staff teams, all in the unavoidable ignorance of the challenges they would encounter. According to Albert Hirschmann's

(1967) Hiding Hand principle, a lack of foresight can be a boon, permitting ambitious challenges to be taken on which only become surmountable through the creativity and resourcefulness of those engaged. Others might argue that what will instead be encountered is a 'Malevolent Hiding Hand' in which misjudgement and optimism bias result in escalating costs, delays, and unanticipated hardships (Flyvbjerg and Sunstein 2016). A substantial research problem is therefore how to assist decision-makers walk the line between ambition and foolhardiness.

How then might managers reach balanced and risk-appropriate decisions under conditions of uncertainty? One approach is to stage investment through small tests of change, experiments and pilot projects, and conditioning further investment on promising results. However any rationalistic approach to staging and scaling a 'best practice' will sit uneasily with a complex model of social innovation which is dynamic, recursive, and provisional involving bricolage and iteration (French et al 2021b). As a compatible alternative, HLS centres the practice of 'Learning as a Management Strategy' in the governance of innovation across multiple system scales. This in turn surfaces new open questions about how roles, governance structures, and cultural dynamics might be configured in response.

Measurement traditionally plays a central role in processes of assurance, particularly in accounting for risk, and accounting for performance and quality of service. Complexity challenges the social convention of relying solely on unified quantitative measures to judge performance and quality of service. Assurance may require seeking a different blend of knowledge. In our opinion, experiential knowledge and qualitative insight, often relegated to the bottom of the scientific hierarchy of evidence, become essential in making policies and programmes relevant and responsive to the dynamic contexts in which they are activated. On the other hand, scientific knowledge based on aggregated statistical evidence may lack local reliability, but could nevertheless inform a more rounded decision-making process when taken in consort with other evidence types. Peer learning environments (Wilson et al 2023) provide an opportunity for collective sense-making of evidence and generating decisions which are both better-informed and better-supported (French 2022). This is an area where 'learning partner' roles might help by introducing critical reflection and challenge, and working to routinise context-informed decision making in uncertainty.

The unintended consequences question

We have described how RTOC-derived approaches have generated a range of counteractive effects and performance paradoxes. The same charge could – and should – be levelled at the complexity-informed approach we offer: what unintended consequences, perverse incentives, and performance paradoxes might a complexity-informed approach generate?

First, it could be that complexity helps the unscrupulous and opportunistic to avoid blame and scrutiny. Bächtold (2021) argues that complexity can shield actors against legitimate demands for accountability and reduce the public's ability to question powerful budget-holders. The bagginess of the term complexity might see problems which are merely complicated or politically contested but ultimately simple, be shepherded into the 'complex' domain in order to excuse inaction. The 2021 report of the Commission on Race and Ethnic Disparities for instance described inequalities in outcomes as resulting from 'unexplained racial disparities', in essence absolving the UK Government's own policies and lack of strategic action from blame.

Complexity could also be used as an intentional obfuscatory device to individualise systemic problems. Critical public health scholarship has documented a 'lifestyle drift' problem where policy focus shifts from preventative 'upstream' contributors to health inequalities toward emphasis on 'downstream' behaviour change. Complexity needs to provoke enthusiasm and motivation to tackle problems rather than subsuming those it engages into a fatalistic rhetoric which 'multiplies rather than solves the complexity burden' (Pawson and Tilley 1997, p 55). Alertness to the potential of such factors seems critical in ensuring the credibility and sustainability of complexity as a constructive basis for public service reform.

The pragmatism question

Effective organisations balance dynamic capabilities with static organisational capacities (Teece et al 1997). The need to develop dynamic capabilities to cope with complexity contends with several key demands on public service professionals, including fulfilling statutory obligations, upholding ethical practice, and prudent budgetary management. How then can the aspirations of dynamic capabilities we outline be reconciled with the practical constraints of contemporary public administration?

Initial moves toward a complexity-informed approach are often made by one or a few transformational leaders, often with external contractor support. The reliance on this small cadre to deliver transformation also risks a lack of resilience as individual leaders move on and contracts end. Recalling W. Edward Deming's famous observation that a bad system will beat a good person every time, there remain significant open questions regarding the methods and supporting infrastructures which can be used to institutionalise dynamic capabilities over the long term.

There should also be care to avoid overstatement and acknowledge the limitations of our theoretical perspective. We acknowledge that many of the interactions between citizens and services should remain transactional – our focus, however, is on the human and relational services. Social outcomes are shaped, held, and experienced directly and immediately by individuals – other outcomes relating to environmental, economic, cultural, or democratic domains of collective wellbeing are not. Our set of dynamic capabilities are substantially reactive and therefore provide limited instruction to help governments and other change agents carry forth anticipatory innovation to respond to predictable, long-term threats. However complex these goals may be, they may require different configurations of dynamic capabilities (Kattel and Mazzucato 2018; Pablo et al 2007).

Rationalism and complexity are two polar 'ideal types', and so inevitably downplay a substantial middleground. Many justify Buurtzorg's place as an exemplar for complexity-engaged working by using a results-based league table to justify its prime position. Plymouth City Council bases its integrated commissioning model on an alliance contract, which is traditionally a results-based contracting approach. Outcome frameworks which blend *both* coercive incentives and soft power approaches to win 'hearts and minds' have been found to perform better than either strategy taken in isolation (French and Wallace 2022). In our experience as learning partners, judgements about performance have been made based on incomplete information, and motivations of others have been questioned. Life and public service reform are full of contradictions.

It may also be that rationalist models can be improved through assessment against dynamic capabilities. A SIB which co-creates its measurement and accountability framework with core partners and operates through relational contracting might develop better dynamic capabilities (see Carter and Ball 2021). However, the incorporation of distinctive logics in such initiatives has been found to polarise in practice, with rationalistic tendencies 'squeezing out' more complexity-appropriate ones (French et al 2022). How blended models of service reform can enhance dynamic capabilities while responding to the structures and logics of rational institutional design seems another significant research area.

The research question

This book has arrived not at a set of directives for practice, but a broad research agenda for the policy and administrative sciences in building complexity-capable public service systems. We consider research a crucial element of a complexity-informed approach to public service reform, ensuring it engages with a broad range of critical voices and wears its tensions and challenges on its sleeve. Our final question is, how can researchers best support a critical, open, and honest engagement with the possibilities and practicalities of complexity-capable public service?

We hope the five questions that have been posed help change-oriented researchers begin to orientate around this agenda. Developing the capability for governing social outcomes is not straightforward, and if managed poorly, may even worsen matters. Informed, robust, and critical research would help a complexity-informed approach to service reform stay honest and reflective about its risks and limitations and provide useful evidence to support a developing practice.

Researchers moving into this space will however confront the same challenges and uncertainties that practitioners face. Academics might productively engage in the broad field of 'action-oriented' research: research approaches which involve both academics and practitioners in boundary-crossing research roles, combining research production and research use *in situ* (French and Hawkins 2020). Associated research methodologies such as action research and action learning, research modalities like co-creation and co-production, and research roles like developmental evaluator, embedded researcher or learning partner provide ample ways in which researchers might play change-oriented roles which also fit the epistemic basis of our theoretical perspective.

Challenging this ambition is a problematic divide between the worlds of academia and practice in the policy and administrative sciences. Academic research played a key role in defining and motivating HLS, but academic engagement in the broader field of complexity-informed policy commentary remains limited. Action-oriented research has played a relatively marginal role in academic scholarship. For example, we found only a handful of papers published in the top six public administration journals over the past 15 years had convincingly utilised methods of Action Research, Action Learning, or Action Inquiry (French and Hawkins 2020). Despite this, with increasing university focus and investment in research impact, knowledge exchange and civic engagement, there is a growing opportunity space to bridge these divides under the common cause of pursuing better social outcomes. Change-oriented researchers within and outwith universities have a crucial role to play in animating and understanding improvement in the issues we discuss in this book. These challenges signal a move within the wider world toward a relational public services stance of which the new approach to outcomes presented in this book is a key element. In order to improve the lives of the communities we live and work in and those we care for this is a change in which we all need to play our part whether we are in our roles as citizens or volunteers, managers or practitioners, policy makers or researchers. We hope the four questions we have posed – alongside the many others we have undoubtedly neglected to consider – provide helpful and motivating guidance for those interested in joining in.

Appendix

Table A.1: HLS narrative case studies

	HLS Narrative Case Studies
1.	Aberlour Child Care Trust
2.	Bicester Healthy New Town
3.	Coast and Vale Community action
4.	Collective Impact Agency
5.	Collective Leadership Scotland
6.	Devon Integrated Health and Social Care
7.	Dorset Health and Social Care
8.	Empowerment
9.	Foreign and Commonwealth Development Office, UK Government
10.	Gateshead Council
11.	Good Cents
12.	GreaterSport
13.	Health Improvement Scotland
14.	Help On Your Doorstep
15.	Here (Care Unbound)
16.	Innovation centre, Finnish National Education Agency (EDUFI)
17.	Lankelly Chase Foundation
18.	Lighthouse Children's Homes
19.	Likewise

(continued)

Table A.1: HLS narrative case studies (continued)

20.	Liverpool City Region Combined Authority
21.	Local Cornerstone
22.	Mayday Trust
23.	Melton Borough Council
24.	Middlesborough Council
25.	Moray Wellbeing Hub
26.	Neighbourhood Midwives
27.	North Devon Pathology Services
28.	Plymouth Alliance
29.	Plymouth Octopus Project
30.	Sobell House Hospice
31.	South Tyneside Alliancing
32.	Stirling Council and The Robertson Trust
33.	Surrey Youth Focus
34.	The Children's Society
35.	The Tudor Trust
36.	Victorian Dept for Education
37.	Vinarice Prison
38.	Wallsend Children's Community
39.	Wellbeing Teams

References

Argyris, C. and Schön, D. (1996) *Organizational Learning II.* Boston: Addison-Wesley.

Argyris, C., Putman, R., Putnam, R.D., and Smith, D.M. (1985) *Action Science (Vol. 13).* San Francisco: Jossey-Bass.

Ashby, W.R. (1956) *An Introduction to Cybernetics.* Oxford: John Wiley and Sons.

Bächtold, S. (2021) 'Donor love will tear us apart: How complexity and learning marginalize accountability in peacebuilding interventions', *International Political Sociology*, 15(4), 504–521. doi:10.1093/ips/olab022.

Badham, R.J. and Sense, A.J. (2006) 'Spiralling up or spinning out: A guide for reflecting on action research practice', *International Journal of Social Research Methodology*, 9(5), 367–377.

Barbrook-Johnson, P. and Penn, A.S. (2022) *Systems Mapping: How to Build and Use Causal Models of Systems.* London: Palgrave Macmillan.

Bennett, H. and Brunner, R. (2022) 'Nurturing the buffer zone: Conducting collaborative action research in contemporary contexts', *Qualitative Research*, 22(1), 74–92.

Bevan, G. and Hood, C. (2006) 'What's measured is what matters: Targets and gaming in the English public health care system', *Public Administration*, 84(3), 517–538.

Bevan, G. and Wilson, D. (2013) 'Does "naming and shaming" work for schools and hospitals? Lessons from natural experiments following devolution in England and Wales', *Public Money & Management*, 33(4), 245–252. https://doi.org/10.1080/09540 962.2013.799801.

Blackmore, C. (2010) *Social Learning Systems and Communities of Practice*. London: Springer.

Blair, T. (1998) *Leading the Way: A New Vision for Local Government*. London: Institute for Public Policy Research.

Blick, A. and Hennessey, P. (2019) *Good Chaps No More: Safeguarding the Constitution in Stressful Times*. London: Constitution Society.

Borgonovi, E., Anessi-Pessina, E., and Bianchi, C. (2018) *Outcome-Based Performance Management in the Public Sector (Vol. 2)*. Cham: Springer.

Boulton, J.G., Allen, P.M., and Bowman, C. (2015) *Embracing Complexity: Strategic Perspectives for an Age of Turbulence*. Oxford: OUP.

Bourne, M., Franco-Santos, M., Micheli, P., and Pavlov, A. (2018) 'Performance measurement and management: A system of systems perspective', *International Journal of Production Research*, 56(8), 2788–2799.

Bovaird, T. (2014) 'Attributing outcomes to social policy interventions – "gold standard" or "fool's gold" in public policy and management?', *Social Policy & Administration*, 48(1), 1–23.

Boydell, T.H. and Blantern, C.J. (2007) 'Action learning as relational practice', *Action Learning: Research and Practice*, 4(1), 95–101.

Boyne, G.A. and Law, J. (2005) 'Setting public service outcome targets: Lessons from local public service agreements', *Public Money & Management*, 25(4), 253–260.

Buchanan, J.M. and Tulloch, G. (1962) *The Calculus of Consent: Logical Foundations of Constitutional Democracy*. Ann Arbor: University of Michigan Press.

Buffardi, A.L., Harvey, B., and Pasanen, T. (2019) '"Learning partners": Overcoming the collective action dilemma of inter-organisational knowledge generation and sharing?', *Development in Practice*, 29(6), 708–722.

Burnes, B., Cooper, C., and West, P. (2003) 'Organisational learning: The new management paradigm?', *Management Decision*, 41(5), 452–464. doi:10.1108/00251740310479304.

Byrne, D. and Callaghan, G. (2014) *Complexity Theory and the Social Sciences: The State of the Art*. London: Routledge.

Carey, G., Malbon, E., Carey, N., Joyce, A., Crammond, B., and Carey, A.G. (2015) 'Systems science and systems thinking for public health: A systematic review of the field', *BMJ Open*, 5(12), e009002. doi:10.1136/bmjopen-2015-009002.

Carter, E. and Ball, N. (2021) 'Spotlighting shared outcomes for social impact programs that work', *Stanford Social Innovation Review*, Available at: https://ssir.org/articles/entry/spotlighting_ shared_outcomes_for_social_impact_programs_that_work# (Accessed 27 September 2021).

Cartwright, N., Bradburn, N.M., and Fuller, J. (2016) 'A theory of measurement', Working Paper. Durham: University of Durham.

Christensen, T. and Lægreid, P. (2007) 'The whole-of-government approach to public sector reform', *Public Administration Review*, 67(6), 1059–1066.

Cilliers, P. (2002) *Complexity and Postmodernism: Understanding Complex Systems*. London: Routledge.

Cornford, J., Wilson, R., Baines, S., and Richardson, R. (2013) 'Local governance in the new information ecology: The challenge of building interpretative communities', *Public Money and Management*, 33(3), 201–208.

Cornford, J. (2019) 'Competing institutional logics of information sharing in public services: Why we often seem to be talking at cross-purposes when we talk about information sharing', *Public Money & Management*, 39(5), 336–345.

Coulson, A. (2009) 'Targets and terror: Government by performance indicators', *Local Government Studies*, 35(2), 271–281. doi:10.1080/03003930902743185.

Cottam, H. (2018) *Radical Help: How We Can Remake the Relationships Between Us and Revolutionise the Welfare State*. London: Hachette UK.

Crossley, S. (2018) *Troublemakers: The Construction of Troubled Families as a Social Problem*. Bristol: Policy Press.

Curtis, S. and Riva, M. (2010) 'Health geographies I: Complexity theory and human health', *Progress in Human Geography*, 34(2), 215–223.

Davidson-Knight, A., Lowe, T., Brossard, M., and Wilson, J. (2017) *A Whole New World: Funding and Commissioning in Complexity*. Newcastle: Collaborate and the University of Newcastle.

Davis, J.H., Schoorman, F.D., and Donaldson, L. (1997) 'Davis, Schoorman, and Donaldson reply: The distinctiveness of agency theory and stewardship theory', *Academy of Management Review*, 22(3), 611.

Department of Health and Social Security. (1980) *Inequalities in Health: Report of a Working Group Chaired by Sir Douglas Black*. Department of Health and Social Security.

Diez Roux, A.V. (2011) 'Complex systems thinking and current impasses in health disparities research', *American Journal of Public Health*, 101(9), 1627–1634.

Dunn, W.N. (2017) *Public Policy Analysis: An Integrated Approach*. 6th edn. New York: Routledge.

DuRose, C. and Richardson, L. (2015) *Designing Public Policy for Co-production: Theory, Practice and Change*. Bristol: Policy Press.

Easterby-Smith, M. (1990) 'Creating a learning organization', *Personnel Review*, 19(5), 24–28.

Eppel, E.A. and Rhodes, M.L. (2018) 'Complexity theory and public management: A "becoming" field', *Public Management Review*, 20(7), 949–959.

Finegood, D.T. (2011) 'The complex systems science of obesity', in J. Cawley (ed) *Handbook of the Social Science of Obesity*. Oxford: Oxford University Press.

Fink, D.S., Keyes, K.M., and Cerdá, M. (2016) 'Social determinants of population health: A systems sciences approach', *Current Epidemiology Reports*, 3(1), 98–105. doi:10.1007/s40471-016-0066-8.

Flyvbjerg, B. and Sunstein, C.R. (2016) 'The principle of the malevolent hiding hand; Or, the planning fallacy writ large', *Social Research*, 83(4), 979–1004.

Franco-Santos, M. and Otley, D. (2018) 'Reviewing and theorizing the unintended consequences of performance management systems', *International Journal of Management Reviews*, 20(3), 696–730.

Freidson, E. (2001) *Professionalism, the Third Logic: On the Practice of Knowledge*. Chicago: University of Chicago Press.

French, M. (2014) 'Achieving outcomes in complex public service environments: the contributions of complex adaptive systems theory', Conference Paper, International Research Conference on Public Management, Birmingham.

French, M. (2017) Achieving Outcomes in Complex Public Service Systems: The Case of the Early Years Collaborative, PhD Thesis. Stirling: University of Stirling. Available at: https://dspace.stir.ac.uk/bitstream/1893/27308/1/Max%20French%20-%20Stirling%20University%20-%20thesis%20final%20version.pdf. (Accessed 12 June 2020).

French, M. (2021) 'Two experiments with outcomes frameworks', *Stanford Social Innovation Review*, 19(4), 57–58. doi:10.48558/bpph-5535.

French, M. (2022) *Evaluation of the Roundtable on Wellbeing in the North of Tyne*. Dunfermline: Carnegie UK Trust.

French, M. and Hawkins, M. (2020) 'The social sciences struggle to be relevant. can action-oriented research help?', *Impact of Social Sciences Blog*. London School of Economics and Political Science. Available at: https://blogs.lse.ac.uk/impactofsocialsciences/ (Accessed 27 April 2021).

French, M. and Lowe, T. (2018) 'The wickedness of public service outcomes: why we need a new public management paradigm', Conference paper, International Research Conference on Public Management, Edinburgh. Available at: https://irspm2018.exordo.com/files/papers/833/final_draft/The_wickedness_of_public_service_outcomes_-_why_we_need_a_new_public_management_paradigm.pdf. (Accessed 10 October 2022).

French, M., Lowe, T., Wilson, R., Rhodes, M.L., and Hawkins, M. (2021a) 'Managing the complexity of outcomes: A new approach to performance measurement and management', in D. Blackman (ed) *Handbook on Performance Management in the Public Sector*. Cheltenham: Edward Elgar Publishing, pp 111–128. https://doi.org/10.4337/9781789901207.00014.

French, M. and Mollinger-Sahba, A. (2021) 'Making performance management relevant in complex and inter-institutional contexts: Using outcomes as performance attractors', *International Journal of Public Sector Management*, 34(3), 377–391. doi:10.1108/IJPSM-03-2020-0071.

French, M., McGowan, K., Rhodes, M. L., and Zivkovic, S. (2021b) 'Advancing the study of complexity in social innovation and social entrepreneurship', *Social Enterprise Journal*, 18(2), 237–251. doi:10.1108/SEJ-05-2022-140.

French, M., Kimmitt, J., Wilson, R., Jamieson, D., and Lowe, T. (2022) 'Social impact bonds and public service reform: Back to the future of New Public Management?', *International Public Management Journal*. doi:10.1080/10967494.2022.2050859.

French, M. and Wallace, J. (2022) 'Performance management for systemic problems: The enabling role of soft power'. Working Paper, Northumbria University. Available at: https://researchportal.northumbria.ac.uk/ws/portalfiles/portal/67951363/Working_paper_performance_management_for_systemic_problems.pdf (Accessed 1 April 2022).

French, M., Wheatman, A., and Hesselgreaves, H. (in press) *Devolved Decision Making*. London: Lankelly Chase Foundation.

Gatrell, A.C. (2005) 'Complexity theory and geographies of health: A critical assessment', *Social Science & Medicine*, 60(12), 2661–2671. doi:10.1016/j.socscimed.2004.11.002.

Gatzweiler, F.W., Reis, S., Zhang, Y., and Jayasinghe, S. (2017) 'Lessons from complexity science for urban health and well-being', *Cities & Health*, 1(2), 210–223. doi:10.1080/23748834.2018.1448551.

Gerrits, L.M. (2012) *Punching Clouds: An Introduction to the Complexity of Public Decision Making*. Litchfield: AZ Emergent.

Gore, A. (1993) *Creating a Government That Works Better & Costs Less: The Report of the National Performance Review: Executive Summary*. US Government Printing Office.

Hallsworth, M. (2011) 'System stewardship. The future of policy making', Working Paper. London: Institute for Government.

Hämäläinen, J. (2015) 'Defining social pedagogy: Historical, theoretical and practical considerations', *The British Journal of Social Work*, 45(3), 1022–1038. doi:10.1093/bjsw/bct174.

Harrison, N. and Geyer, R. (2022) *Governing Complexity in the 21st Century*. London: Routledge.

Hatton, K. (2013) *Social Pedagogy in the UK: Theory and Practice*. Lyme Regis: Russell House Publishing Ltd.

Hawk, T.F. and Zand, D.E. (2014) 'Parallel organization: Policy formulation, learning, and interdivision integration', *The Journal of Applied Behavioral Science*, 50(3), 307–336.

Haynes, P. (2015) *Managing Complexity in the Public Services*. 2nd edn. London: Routledge.

Heifetz, R.A., Grashow, A., and Linksy, M. (2009) *The Practice of Adaptive Leadership: Tools and Tactics for Changing Your Organization and the World*. Cambridge, MA: Harvard Business Press.

Heinrich, C.J. (2002) 'Outcomes-based performance management in the public sector: Implications for government accountability and effectiveness', *Public Administration Review*, 62(6), 712–725.

Hernandez, M. (2012) 'Toward an understanding of the psychology of stewardship', *Academy of Management Review*, 37(2), 172–193.

Hesselgreaves, H., French, M., Hawkins, M., Lowe, T., Wheatman, A., Martin, M., and Wilson, R. (2021) 'New development: The emerging role of a "learning partner" relationship in supporting public service reform', *Public Money & Management*, 41(7), 573–576. https://doi.org/10.1080/09540962.2021.1909274.

Heydecker, R., Ormston, H., and Wallace, J. (2022) *GDWe: A Spotlight on Democratic Wellbeing*. Dunfermline: Carnegie UK Trust.

Hirschman, A.O. (1967) 'The principle of the hiding hand', *The Public Interest* (Winter): 10–23.

Hobbs, C. (2019) *Systemic Leadership for Local Governance: Tapping the Resource Within*. London: Palgrave Macmillan Cham.

Hood, C. (1991) 'A public management for all seasons?' *Public Administration*, 69(1), 3–19. doi:10.1111/j.1467-9299.1991.tb00779.x.

Hood, C. and Dixon, R. (2016) 'Not what it said on the tin? Reflections on three decades of UK Public Management Reform', *Financial Accountability & Management*, 32(4), 409–428. doi:10.1111/faam.12095.

Jackson, M.C. (2019) *Critical Systems Thinking and the Management of Complexity*. Hoboken, NJ: John Wiley & Sons.

Jakobsen, M.L., Baekgaard, M., Moynihan, D.P., and van Loon, N. (2018) 'Making sense of performance regimes: Rebalancing external accountability and internal learning', *Perspectives on Public Management and Governance*, 1(2), 127–141. doi:10.1093/ppmgov/gvx001.

James, S. (1993) 'The idea brokers: The impact of think tanks on British government', *Public Administration*, 71(4), 491–506. doi:10.1111/j.1467-9299.1993.tb00988.x.

Jamieson, D., Wilson, R., Martin, M., Lowe, T., Kimmitt, J., Gibbon, J., and French, M. (2020) 'Data for outcome payments or information for care? A sociotechnical analysis of the management information system in the implementation of a social impact bond', *Public Money & Management*, 40(3), 213–224. doi:10.1080/09540962.2020.1714306.

Jayasinghe, S. (2011) 'Conceptualising population health: From mechanistic thinking to complexity science', *Emerging Themes in Epidemiology*, 8(1), 1–7.

Jayasinghe, S. (2015) 'Social determinants of health inequalities: Towards a theoretical perspective using systems science', *International Journal for Equity in Health*, 14(1), 1–8.

Jensen, M.C. and Meckling, W.H. (1976) 'Theory of the firm: Managerial behavior, agency costs and ownership structure', *Journal of Financial Economics*, 3(4), 305–360.

Johnson, G. and Leavitt, W. (2001) 'Building on success: Transforming organizations through an appreciative inquiry', *Public Personnel Management*, 30(1), 129–136.

Kaplan, R.S. and Norton, D.P. (2015) *Balanced Scorecard Success: The Kaplan-Norton Collection (4 Books)*. Cambridge, MA: Harvard Business Review Press.

Kattel, R. and Mazzucato, M. (2018) 'Mission-oriented innovation policy and dynamic capabilities in the public sector', *Industrial and Corporate Change*, 27(5), 787–801.

Kemmis, S., McTaggart, R., and Nixon, R. (2014) 'Introducing Critical Participatory Action Research', in S. Kemmis, R. McTaggart, and R. Nixon (eds) *The Action Research Planner: Doing Critical Participatory Action Research*. London: Springer, pp 1–31. https://doi.org/10.1007/978-981-4560-67-21.

Kuhn, T. (1962) *The Structure of Scientific Revolutions*. 2nd edn. Chicago: University of Chicago Press.

Kurtz, C.F. and Snowden, D.J. (2003) 'The new dynamics of strategy: Sense-making in a complex and complicated world', *IBM Systems Journal*, 42(3), 462–483. doi:10.1147/sj.423.0462.

Lave, J. and Wenger, E. (1991) *Situated Learning: Legitimate Peripheral Participation*. Cambridge: Cambridge University Press.

Lent, A. and Studdert, J. (2019) 'The community paradigm: why public services need radical change and how it can be achieved', New Local Government Network. Available at: www.newlocal. org.uk/wp-content/uploads/2019/03/The-Community-Parad igm_New-Local-2.pdf (Accessed 10 March 2022).

Lipsky, M. (1971) 'Street-level bureaucracy and the analysis of urban reform', *Urban Affairs Quarterly*, 6, 392–409.

Lowe, T. (2013) 'New development: The paradox of outcomes – the more we measure, the less we understand', *Public Money & Management*, 33(3), 213–216.

Lowe, T., French, M., and Hawkins, M. (2020a) 'Navigating complexity: The future of public service', in H. Sullivan, H. Dickinson, and H. Henderson (eds) *The Palgrave Handbook of the Public Servant*. Cham: Springer International Publishing, pp 1–19. doi:10.1007/978-3-030-03008-7_16-1.

Lowe, T., French, M. and Hawkins, M. (2020b) 'The Human, Learning, Systems approach to commissioning in complexity', in A. Bonner (ed) *Local Authorities and the Social Determinants of Health*. Bristol: Bristol University Press, pp 241–262.

Lowe, T., French, M., Hawkins, M., Hesselgreaves, H. and Wilson, R. (2021a) 'Responding to complexity in public services – the human learning systems approach', *Public Money & Management*, 41(7), 573–576. doi:10.1080/09540962.2020.1832738.

Lowe, T., Brogan, A., Eichsteller, G., Hawkins, M., Hesselgreaves, H., Plimmer, D., and Terry, V., et al (2021b) *Human Learning Systems: Public Service for the Real World*. Allithwaite: United Kingdom: ThemPra Social Pedagogy. https://realworld.report/ (Accessed 10 June 2022).

Lowe, T. and French, M. (2018) 'The meaning of evidence in a complexity-informed public management', in Health Foundation, *A Recipe for Action: Using Wider Evidence for a Healthier UK*. London: Health Foundation. Available at: www.health.org.uk/ publications/a-recipe-for-action-using-wider-evidence-for-a-healthier-uk (Accessed 10 July 2020).

Lowe, T. and Wilson, R. (2017) 'Playing the game of outcomes-based performance management. Is gamesmanship inevitable? Evidence from theory and practice', *Social Policy & Administration*, 51(7), 981–1001.

Lowe, T., Wilson, R., and Boobis, S. (2016) 'The Performance Management of Complex Systems – Enabling Adaptation', Conference Paper, Performance Management Association Conference, April 2016.

Lowe, T., Padmanabhan, C., McCart, D., McNeill, K., Brogan, A., and Smith, M. (2022) *Human Learning Systems: A Practical Guide for the Curious*. Centre for Public Impact. https://www.centrefor publicimpact.org/assets/pdfs/hls-practical-guide.pdf (Accessed 10 October 2022).

Lowe, T. and Plimmer, D. (2019) *Exploring the New World: Practical Insights for Funding, Commissioning and Managing in Complexity*. Newcastle: Newcastle Business School and Collaborate CIC.

Marmot, M. and Wilkinson, R. (2005) *Social Determinants of Health*. Oxford: Oxford University Press.

McLoughlin, I. and Wilson, R. (2013) *Digital Government at Work: A Social Informatics Perspective*. Oxford: Oxford University Press.

Melnyk, S.A., Bititci, U., Platts, K., Tobias, J., and Andersen, B. (2014) 'Is performance measurement and management fit for the future?', *Management Accounting Research*, 25(2), 173–186. doi:10.1016/j.mar.2013.07.007.

Mickan, S. and Coates, D. (2022) 'Embedded researchers' purpose and practice: Current perspectives from Australia', *The International Journal of Health Planning and Management*, 37(1), 133–142.

Miller, E. (2014) 'Considering two outcomes paradigms: The improving (person-centred) and the proving (managerialist) agendas', in Hessel, S. (ed) *Human Rights and Social Equality: Challenges for Social Work*. Farnham: Ashgate Publishing, pp 34–39.

Mintzberg, H. and Waters, J.A. (1985) 'Of strategies, deliberate and emergent', *Strategic Management Journal*, 6(3), 257–272. doi:10.1002/smj.4250060306.

Moore, M.H. (1995) *Creating Public Value: Strategic Management in Government*. Cambridge, MA: Harvard University Press.

Morin, E. (2006) 'Restricted complexity, general complexity. Science and us: Philosophy and Complexity', *Singapore: World Scientific*, 1–25.

Mowles, C. and Norman, K. (eds) (2022) *Complexity and the Public Sector*. London: Taylor & Francis.

Muir, R. (2014) 'The relational state: Beyond marketisation and managerialism', *Juncture*, 20(4), 280–286. https://doi.org/10.1111/j.2050-5876.2014.00766.x.

New System Alliance (2020) *Wisdom from the System*. Available at: https://newsystemalliance.org/wp-content/uploads/2020/12/Wisdom-from-the-System.pdf (Accessed 10 June 2022).

Needham, C. and Mangan, C. (2016) 'The 21st-century public servant: Working at three boundaries of public and private', *Public Money & Management*, 36(4), 265–272. https://doi.org/10.1080/09540962.2016.1162592.

Needham, C., Mastracci, S., and Mangan, C. (2017) 'The emotional labour of boundary spanning', *Journal of Integrated Care*, 25(4), 288–300. doi:10.1108/JICA-04-2017-0008.

Osborne, D. and Gaebler, T. (1992) *Reinventing Government*. New York: Addison-Wesley Publishing Co.

Osborne S.P. (ed) (2010) *The New Public Governance? Emerging Perspectives on the Theory and Practice of Public Governance.* London: Routledge.

Pablo, A.L., Reay, T., Dewald, J.R., and Casebeer, A.L. (2007) 'Identifying, enabling and managing dynamic capabilities in the public sector', *Journal of Management Studies*, 44(5), 687–708.

Panchamia, N. and Thomas, P. (2014) 'Public service agreements and the prime minister's delivery unit', *Institute for Government*. https://www.instituteforgovernment.org.uk/sites/default/files/case%20study%20psas.pdf (Accessed 10 June 2022).

Pawson, R. and Tilley, N. (1997) *Realistic Evaluation*. London: SAGE.

Pearce, N. and Merletti, F. (2006) 'Complexity, simplicity, and epidemiology', *International Journal of Epidemiology*, 35(3), 515–519.

Pell, C., Wilson, R. and Lowe, T. (eds) (2016) *Kittens Are Evil: Little Heresies in Public Policy*. Axminster: Triarchy Press.

Pell, C., Wilson, R., Lowe, T. and Myers J. (eds) (2020) *Kittens Are Evil 2: Little Heresies in Public Policy*. Axminster: Triarchy Press.

Perrin, B. (2007) 'Moving from outputs to outcomes: Practical advice from governments around the world', in J.D. Breul and C. Moravitz (eds) *Integrating Performance and Budgets: The Budget Office of Tomorrow*. Plymouth, England: Rowman & Littlefield, pp 107–168.

Perry, J.L., Hondeghem, A., and Wise, L.R. (2010) 'Revisiting the motivational bases of public service: Twenty years of research and an agenda for the future', *Public Administration Review*, 70(5), 681–690.

Phelps, R. and Hase, S. (2002) 'Complexity and action research: Exploring the theoretical and methodological connections', *Educational Action Research*, 10(3), 507–524. doi:10.1080/09650790200200198.

Piening, E.P. (2013) 'Dynamic capabilities in public organizations', *Public Management Review*, 15(2), 209–245. doi:10.1080/14719037.2012.708358.

Piggot-Irvine, E., Rowe, W., and Ferkins, L. (2015) 'Conceptualizing indicator domains for evaluating action research', *Educational Action Research*, 23(4), 545–566. doi:10.1080/09650792.2015.1042984.

Pollitt, C., Harrison, S., Dowswell, G., Jerak-Zuiderent, S., and Bal, R. (2010) 'Performance regimes in health care: Institutions, critical junctures and the logic of escalation in England and the Netherlands', *Evaluation*, 16(1), 13–29. doi:10.1177/1356389009350026.

Pollitt, C. and Bouckaert, G. (2017) *Public Management Reform: A Comparative Analysis into the Age of Austerity*. Oxford: Oxford University Press.

Pollitt, C. (2013) 'The evolving narratives of public management reform', *Public Management Review*, 15(6), 899–922. doi:10.1080/14719037.2012.725761.

Porter, T. (1986) *The Rise of Statistical Thinking 1820–1900*. Princeton, NJ: Princeton University Press.

Radin, B.A. (2006) *Challenging the Performance Movement: Accountability, Complexity, and Democratic Values*. Washington, DC Georgetown University Press.

Reason, P. and Torbert, W. (2001) 'The action turn: Toward a transformational social science', *Concepts and Transformation*, 6(1), 1–37. doi:10.1075/cat.6.1.02rea.

Revans, R.W. (1982) 'What is Action Learning?', *Journal of Management Development*, 1(3), 64–75. doi.org/10.1108/eb051529.

Rhodes, R.A. (1997) *Understanding Governance: Policy Networks, Governance, Reflexivity and Accountability*. Berkshire: Open University.

Romzek, B. and Dubnick, M. (1987) 'Accountability in the public sector: Lessons from the Challenger tragedy', *Public Administration Review*, 47, 227–238. doi:10.2307/975901.

Rutter, H., Savona, N., Glonti, K., Bibby, J., Cummins, S., and Finegood, D.T., et al (2017) 'The need for a complex systems model of evidence for public health', *The Lancet*, 390(10112), 2602–2604.

Schedler, K. and Proeller, I. (2010) *Outcome-oriented Public Management: A Responsibility-based Approach to the New Public Management*. Charlotte, NC: IAP.

Schensul, J.J. (2009) 'Community, culture and sustainability in multilevel dynamic systems intervention science', *American Journal of Community Psychology*, 43(3), 241–256. doi:10.1007/s10464-009-9228-x.

Senge, P. (1990) *The Fifth Discipline: The Art and Practice of the Learning Organization*. New York: Doubleday.

Simon, H.A. (1957) *Administrative Behaviour*. 2nd edn. New York: Macmillan.

Sinclair, J. (1798) *The Statistical Account of Scotland* (21 vol). Edinburgh: William Creech.

Smith, M. and Bititci, U.S. (2017) 'Interplay between performance measurement and management, employee engagement and performance', *International Journal of Operations & Production Management*, 37, 1207–1228.

Smith, M. (2020) 'The tangled and the trapped', blog. Available at: https://collaboratecic.com/the-tangled-and-the-trapped-d702d023bcb2. (Accessed 22 January 2021).

Smyth, J. and Dow, A. (1998) 'What's wrong with outcomes? Spotter planes, action plans, and steerage of the educational workplace', *British Journal of Sociology of Education*, 19(3), 291–303. doi:10.1080/0142569980190302.

Soss, J., Fording, R., and Schram, S.F. (2011) 'The organization of discipline: From performance management to perversity and punishment', *Journal of Public Administration Research and Theory*, 21(suppl_2), i203–i232. doi:10.1093/jopart/muq095.

Stake, R.E. (1995) *The Art of Case Study Research*. Thousand Oaks, CA: Sage.

Sterman, J.D. (2002) 'All models are wrong: Reflections on becoming a systems scientist', *System Dynamics Review*, 18(4), 501–531. doi:10.1002/sdr.261.

Teece, D.J., Pisano, G., and Shuen, A. (1997) 'Dynamic capabilities and strategic management', *Strategic Management Journal*, 18(7), 509–533.

Uhl-Bien, M., Marion, R., and McKelvey, B. (2007) 'Complexity leadership theory: Shifting leadership from the industrial age to the knowledge era', *The Leadership Quarterly*, 18(4), 298–318.

Van de Ven, A.H. (2007) *Engaged Scholarship: A Guide for Organizational and Social Research*. Oxford: OUP on Demand.

Van Thiel, S. and Leeuw, F.L. (2002) 'The performance paradox in the public sector', *Public Performance & Management Review*, 25(3), 267–281.

Vandenbroeck, P., Goossens, J., and Clemens, M. (2007) *Tackling Obesities: Future Choices—Building the Obesity System Map*. Government Office for Science. Available at: https://assets.pub lishing.service.gov.uk/government/uploads/system/uploads/atta chment_data/file/295154/07-1179-obesity-building-system-map.pdf. (Accessed 10 June 2022).

Vindrola-Padros, C., Eyre, L., Baxter, H., Cramer, H., George, B., and Wye, L., et al (2019) 'Addressing the challenges of knowledge co-production in quality improvement: Learning from the implementation of the researcher-in-residence model', *BMJ Quality & Safety*, 28(1), 67–73. doi:10.1136/bmjqs-2017-007127.

Wallace, J. (2019) *Wellbeing and Devolution: Reframing the Role of Government in Scotland, Wales and Northern Ireland*. London: Palgrave Macmillan.

Weick, K.E. (1976) 'Educational organizations as loosely coupled systems', *Administrative Science Quarterly*, 21(1), 1–19. https://doi.org/10.2307/2391875.

WHO (2008) *Closing the Gap in a Generation: Health Equity Through Action On the Social Determinants of Health: Final Report of the Commission on Social Determinants of Health*. Geneva: World Health Organization.

Wilson, L.C., Hawkins, M., French, M., Lowe, T., and Hesselgreaves, H. (2023) 'Learning communities: An approach to dismantling barriers to collective improvement', *Public Money & Management*. doi: 10.1080/09540962.2022.2116179

Wilson, R., Baines, S., Hardill, I., and Ferguson, M. (2013) 'Editorial: Information for local governance. Data is the solution … what was the question again?', *Public Money & Management*, 33(3), 163–166.

Wilson, R., Cornford, J., Baines, S., and Mawson, J. (2011) 'Information for localism? Policy sensemaking for local governance', *Public Money & Management*, 31(4), 295–300.

Wilson, W. (1887) 'The study of administration', *Political Science Quarterly*, 2(2), 197–222.

Wimbush, E. (2011) 'Implementing an outcomes approach to public management and accountability in the UK – are we learning the lessons?', *Public Money & Management*, 31(3), 211–218. doi:10.1080/09540962.2011.573237.

Zuber-Skerritt, O. (2002) 'A model for designing action learning and action research programs', *The Learning Organization*, 9(4), 143–149.

Index

References to figures appear in *italic* type;
those in **bold** type refer to tables.